THE PATIENT REVOLUTION

of related interest

Values in Health and Social Care
An Introductory Workbook
Ray Sumuriwo, Ben Hannigan, Stephen Pattison and Andrew Todd
ISBN 978 1 78592 063 9
eISBN 978 1 78450 320 8

Observation in Health and Social Care
Applications for Learning, Research and
Practice with Children and Adults
Edited by Helen Hingley-Jones, Clare Parkinson and Lucille Allain
ISBN 978 1 84905 675 5
eISBN 978 1 78450 181 5

Whistleblowing and Ethics in Health and Social Care
Angie Ash
ISBN 978 1 84905 632 8
eISBN 978 1 78450 108 2

Integrated Care in Action
A Practical Guide for Health, Social Care and Housing Support
Robin Miller, Hilary Brown and Catherine Mangan
ISBN 978 1 84905 646 5
eISBN 978 1 78450 142 6

How We Treat the Sick
Neglect and Abuse in Our Health Services
Michael Mandelstam
ISBN 978 1 84905 160 6
eISBN 978 0 85700 355 3

Emerging Values in Health Care
The Challenge for Professionals
Edited by Stephen Pattison, Ben Hannigan, Roisin Pill and Huw Thomas
ISBN 978 1 84310 947 1
eISBN 978 0 85700 365 2

THE PATIENT REVOLUTION

How We Can Heal the
Healthcare System

David Gilbert

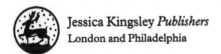

Jessica Kingsley *Publishers*
London and Philadelphia

First published in 2020
by Jessica Kingsley Publishers
73 Collier Street
London N1 9BE, UK
and
400 Market Street, Suite 400
Philadelphia, PA 19106, USA

www.jkp.com

Library of Congress Cataloging in Publication Data
A CIP catalog record for this book is available from the Library of Congress

British Library Cataloguing in Publication Data
A CIP catalogue record for this book is available from the British Library

ISBN 978 1 78592 538 2
eISBN 978 1 78450 932 3

Printed and bound in Great Britain

For Susan – For your patience, encouragement, advice and love. This book would not be without you

For Samuel and Adam – For the hope and love you have brought to my life and writing

CONTENTS

But Much Is

It is hard to avoid the difficulty of sadness
whilst listening long-distance
to another's song

as when strangers curve into each other's
unlikely bodies, whiteness
of mute swans

muttering quietly, then mirroring a heart.
Indistinguishably apart.
But much is

to do with that sorrowful, thin, brightly lit
stuttering attention. Pain
is what binds love.

David Gilbert

PREFACE

The Tale of the Jewel Merchants

Those of us unfortunate, weakened, damaged and fallen from grace were banished to the harsh and arid Valley of Despair.

There, we crawled alone to find caves in which we could live our days and suffer through the cold nights.

We were changed, frightened and alone. What we had hoped to be, we could no longer be. What we could do, we could no longer do. Who we were, was no longer who we would be. We were refugees of mind, body and land.

Those of us that survived – many did not – did the best we could.

We eked out a life in the harsh terrain. We learned to be creative to survive the everyday bleakness – to forage for sparse and strange plants that bore orange bitter fruit, to bear the twists of our cruel minds that woke us at 3am to the bloody cries of wolves. And to do the best we could to adjust to the terrible blackness of the cave that was now our home.

Over the snail-like years, we came to explore the depths of our caves. We discovered broken stones around us – in the walls, around us on the floor. Our very brokenness led us to delve into broken things around us – we yearned for connection, with ourselves, with others, with stones, with the world.

Some of us started tunnelling. Some strange force kept us going, and kept us digging, exploring. We began excavating under the floors of the cave and unearthed more luminous and reflective objects. We could only go deeper.

We began to polish the stones and were amazed to discover that the act of polishing changed their colour, they became reflective – we saw our own true faces for the first time in years – shaded in amazing hues of violet and gold. We glowed.

Maybe, after all, there had been something wrong, not with us but the world around us.

Perhaps the banished had a story to tell, maybe we had found something secret that we needed to share. Could the jewels be precious to others, and not just us? If only the market dwellers in the citadels would see what we had to bring, then everything might change.

A few of us set off from our caves, excited and terrified. But our legs were weak, and our carts rickety. We were not able to get far. The heaviness of our load was almost unbearable, the horses we tried to harness would not pull in the right direction. There was no support from strangers.

What kept us going? I am still unsure. We did not know

where we were going precisely. The roads had changed. They seemed to loop around on each other. They were bumpy and led by treacherous ravines and up bleak hillsides.

Oh the many times we almost gave up! We fell into telling each other things would never change. And a few tried to get back to their caves, or threw out the jewels from their cart, despising their abhorrent erstwhile dreams as nightmares or fantasies.

And then, one night, we camped close to a river. And a few of us fell to telling our tales and shared them under an elm tree. And more and more of us came – it was like magic.

We could see that the market dwellers needed us as much as or perhaps even more than we needed them.

I wish I knew the ending of this tale. Many of us are still isolated and alone. A few of us have managed to set up stall and a few of us have exchanged our jewels – albeit at a lower price than their true value.

It is not easy. But every time we meet, we feel stronger. And our jewels glow more brightly. The Jewel Merchants are journeying as we speak. Let the jewels be shared.

INTRODUCTION

On a cold, rainy day seven years ago, Alison Cameron, Michael Seres and I travelled from Waterloo Station to meet Anya de Iongh (now Patient Editor at the *British Medical Journal*) in the basement of a Winchester cafe. We talked for hours about what it was like to live with illness and why we were crazy enough to think our work might one day be worthwhile – not just for us, but for several thousand other dreamers.

We had chosen a bizarre career route after being ill – not to curl up and do what sensible people should (i.e. heal), but go back into the fray and try to change the healthcare system. We saw clearly *what* was good and bad about it. We saw clearly *who* was good and bad. We saw clearly *where* it was good and bad. We had not been blinded by pain; our eyes had been opened to what healthcare was like.

We could help – we wanted to help

I've had thousands of cups of coffees with others since then – those people we then started to call 'patient leaders'. That is: people affected by life-changing illness who want to change the lives of others of our ilk. Or: people who have been through stuff, who know stuff, who want to change stuff. Or, more poetically: those who 'bring jewels of wisdom and insight from the caves of suffering'.

We are still here. Sometimes hanging on with our fingernails. Sometimes on the decision-making stage with the bigwigs. Many times crying in the toilets. Mostly fluttering in between, as well as relapsing.

On the whole, despite our wanting to help and knowing we can, we are habitually prevented from doing so by a system that has, until recently, not valued what we bring. This book is about what we have learned at personal and professional levels along the crazy path we have taken. And, we are learning how to breach the wall of the citadels and change the way the healthcare fortress works.

Or, let's use the language in a less combative way: we are equalising spaces and power, becoming true partners with other system leaders. After all, everyone in healthcare wants the same thing, surely?

We can help. We know intimately what it is like to feel vulnerable and powerless, the effect of pain and suffering on lives, the primacy of healing relationships in care and what good and poor services look like. This combination of vision, humanity and integrity are essential components of high-quality leadership.

Over my 30-year career in patient and public engagement, I have discovered the excitement of what 'patient voices' could bring. But also the frustrations of a National Health Service (NHS) systematically unable to value people like us.

How we can help

Having patients as partners in the room means looking at problems differently. If you get a bunch of doctors and nurses talking about why people don't turn up for appointments, the likelihood is that they will focus on people needing to take more responsibility. Or they will say we should use text reminders. Fine.

But what if it is about inflexible appointment systems, people having too much pain to negotiate buses or the bus stops being too far away from the surgery? Having patients who know about real access issues changes the discussion. It draws attention to who is not in the room, including the local authority, for example.

Focusing properly on what matters to patients can only be done if patients are part of decisions. It leads to 'pathway redesign', aka changing what we do (let's try and avoid the coarsening effects of corporate-speak). It leads to better awareness of how people get to places and when (access issues), information and explanations needed at each stage, more humanity and better customer care.

Patient engagement also promotes the finding of potential solutions to problems. Patients have the passion, insight, imagination and freedom from institutionally limited thinking to ask 'What if...?' They also widen the array of options for improvement and change.

This process changes relationships. With patients in the room, others are given permission to explore. Dynamics change, trusted relationships develop, people work together and move beyond us–them conversations to dialogue. Shared decision-making emerges. Power shifts.

One woman came up to me after a focus group and said, 'Can you stop using the word "discharge" as if I am effluent or snot to be got rid of? That is all about your efficiency targets. For me, it is about "coming home".'

The conversation then focused on what it feels like when you come home from an operation or how it feels when someone says you are discharged. We saw it from the point of view of who used the service, not through an institutional lens that had a blind spot. How does it feel to be ejected, alone, still in pain, unused to being back in the community, perhaps without support? Not only was this a more 'patient-centred conversation', but the social workers and district nurses around the table started to chip in because they could see the problem – it was about everybody working together.

There are also individual benefits to good engagement. Patients feel more confident, develop new skills and build on those skills buried during times of illness – and come to feel better. All those featured in this book and thousands of others who have been robbed of their identities and capabilities want to unlock their potential once again. They need to restore their professional and human confidence.

Recently, in my work in Sussex, we interviewed people for 'patient partner' roles. One said of the information for applicants: 'I was gobsmacked. I have never been asked what I have learned during this period of pain and suffering, let alone someone asking me to bring those skills to the table. It is obvious, isn't it? Why can't the NHS see that we are people still, that illness has not robbed us of our intelligence?'

Staff gain too. Morale is lifted as conversations become about what can be done; they can feel that we are truly all in this together. This sort of work rehumanises healthcare. Time and time again, I have seen health professionals light up when patients talk about themselves in a way that sparks discussion on what it is like to be ill and what matters. And, what could be improved.

Not only are conversations quickly brought down to earth by people who cannot – will not – use jargon, but patients provide permission for the barriers to come down. For professionals, this can reconnect them with the passion they have for healing – why they came into the realm of service in the first place.

The result is better-quality decisions. If people know why decisions have been made and have been part of that process, this generates trust and confidence, and it becomes easier to build consensus.

I was once part of a mental health 'blue-sky' thinking exercise. We were asked to imagine how many community mental health teams we wanted in our area. 'As many as possible – eight?' I said. The finance director broke rank, bless him. 'We can afford two at most. This blue-sky thinking stuff is BS. Let's be honest and have proper discussions. We in the management team are just scared of having grown-up discussions with service users.'

We hated him for five minutes. Then we realised that this is what we wanted and valued as service users – straight talk, honest, authentic, vulnerable. For the rest of the day, we talked about thresholds and how ill you had to be to get into the service, and what happens to those left behind. We designed ways of supporting people.

Difficult discussions. But unavoidable. I think patients and communities are ready. If we continue to hide in obfuscation and the institutional fear that lies at the heart of impenetrable guff in documents, then we are all losers. And the anger will mount.

Decision-making is being made by stealth and in secret, partly because of fear about grown-up conversations. Yet managers go on courses about collaborative leadership and are encouraged to be 'authentic'. The tension between that and what they find when they come back to the ranch is stark. They go back to find behind-closed-doors discussions about targets and mysterious policy pronouncements about 'new models of care' (which are not discussed early on and openly with communities).

I believe that discussions about the very future of the NHS are being had right now by a small cartel of policy makers – a collective of hunched shoulders, lowered eyes, whispered voices, whose decisions get sieved through the corporate communications machine and end up as impenetrable gobbledygook. Nobody knows what the hell is really going on. In my opinion, and in my experience, fear of grown-up conversations with us, the punters, is at the root of stealth-like changes to the NHS.

True patient partnership then would have deep implications for transparency, governance and accountability. At local level, I have seen and heard about dozens of changes in policy and practice as a result of patients being partners in improvement work: making guidelines more flexible, better ways to tackle access and equalities, tackling attitudes and behaviours, different ways of meeting unmet need – the list is endless.

One service found that people weren't turning up for scans. So they spent £10,000 on leaflets reminding people of why scans were a good thing. And saying that if people did not turn up they would go to the back of the waiting list. I was in the room with the head nurse when one of her colleagues came rushing in saying, 'We've got it all wrong.' They had found that most of those who had not turned up were scared of going into the machine. So they talked with patients and changed things – music, soft lighting, better explanations of what would happen... Voila.

There are even benefits beyond the project. When people see the advantages of patients as partners for improvement and change in one area, they will help spread it to others. It is a virtuous cycle with implications for scaling up improvement processes, spreading good practice and sustainability. I have seen neurologists come into great diabetes conversations between patients and staff, and think, 'OK, I will try that in my team.'

It could help heal the NHS at so many levels.

What stops us

But for all this to happen, we must change traditional approaches to involving or engaging patients. They do not work, and so we fail to value the jewels offered or to change the 'currency' of healthcare toward what matters.

Patient and public engagement, as traditionally conceived, buffers power by distancing patients from decision-making. Thus, it maintains the status quo by preserving the institutional authority of professional system leaders. Ironically, when engagement is seen to fail, as it often does, this can be attributed to the lack of value that patients bring rather than to faulty mechanisms. The engagement industry focuses largely on inputs, activities and processes (the methods of gathering data, how to capture views, etc.) over impact and outcomes.

The approaches and methods used rely on two main styles. The first is that of feedback: patients are invited to fill in questionnaires, attend focus groups or tell their stories (if they are lucky) at board meetings or the like. The focus is what happened to them in the past, and mostly on their experience of services (rather than living with a condition or their lives beyond the institutional scope of interest), and the meaning of their data is left to professionals to assess through their own lenses based on their own assumptions and often narrow, institutionalised thinking (often what is seen as feasible rather than necessary).

Patients are not permitted to eyeball the data or bring their own interpretations to it, let alone be partners in decisions about what to do. This feedback approach mirrors traditional medical paternalistic models – you tell us the symptoms and we will provide the diagnosis and treatment. It is stuck in child–parent mode.

The second style is scrutiny. Whenever there is a governance committee, an advisory group or the like, the call goes out for a lay representative. I know a patient and public involvement lead who likened her role to that of 'lay rep pimp'. Without clarity of role, support or training, a representative is expected to bring the patient perspective to the decision-making table.

I was once asked, 'So David, what do patients think?' 'What, all of them?' I thought. In search of credibility, and leaning on what we know, we tell our stories, and half the people in the room applaud this 'telling truth to power' and the other half fall asleep ('Another patient with an axe to grind,' or 'Personal agenda,' they mutter later in the corridors). If we wise up and come to the table next time wearing a suit and tie, brandishing data, those who were awake last time fall asleep and accuse us of 'going native'. I have written about this representative trap in more detail elsewhere.

The consequence of failed representational mechanisms is that committees lapse into a default 'us-and-them' mode. Frustrated, marginalised and unprepared representatives start finger-wagging or fall silent. This is adolescent–parent-style engagement. If we are serious about partnership, we need to overhaul the engagement industry.

Patient leaders (and, of course, carers) can have many roles though, not just in 'patient and public engagement'. Some are entrepreneurs. Others are campaigners or activists, online dialogue specialists or improvement advisors, or they help organisations as governors or are part of inspection processes. They work at local, regional and national levels. But the overall direction is the same: to change health and healthcare, to reap the benefits of our wisdom and expertise.

Meanwhile, the system, on the whole, still refuses to value us for what we bring. This at a time when the call is for integration, collaborative working and innovation. Instead of turning to us for help and advice, the NHS seems to glory in restructuring itself and an endless recycling of top leaders and empty rhetoric about 'putting patients at the heart of care'.

We know there needs to be wider investment in skills development; indeed, one might question why tens of millions of pounds is spent investing in the capabilities of managerial and clinical leadership and none on this emerging army of people who could – and I think will – regenerate healthcare.

There is still a widespread assumption that system leaders are professionals, but for patient leaders to achieve their full potential, they also need the learning and development that enables them to be true leaders.

This is what Mark Doughty and I did by creating the Centre for Patient Leadership (CPL) in 2012: to support patients and carers to be influential change agents working in partnership with others. This built on our inventing the notion of patient leaders/patient leadership two years previously.

CPL trained several hundred patients and carers to develop the capabilities to work with professionals as equal partners. Further information on patient leadership is available online at: www.inhealthassociates.co.uk/patient-leadership-articles-and-reports.

However, there has to be an equal emphasis on creating the right opportunities, for example in governance, research and audit, service improvement and training and education. This could be at a local or national level but needs to be where professionals are willing and able to work as partners too.

Opportunities must also be created at a senior level. It is not right that a service purporting to deliver 'women-centred care' is led entirely by men. In a few years' time, it will seem odd that we have ever had a patient-centred NHS run entirely by clinical and managerial leaders.

And the excuses made for not working with us continue to do the rounds: having patients involved will take too long, slow us down, not yield benefit. That patients are too demanding, negative, angry and expectant, and their demands will be unachievable, or, conversely, too passive, their views unsurprising (oh, we knew that already).

People's legitimacy and role is questioned – they are not representative and may have an 'axe to grind' or, conversely, they will become co-opted and become the 'usual suspects'.

Having seen true patient leadership and real patient partnership challenge all these myths, it is hard to avoid the conclusion that this is mostly about power.

Meanwhile, the work is largely unsupported. We do not have a 'royal college' or any kind of infrastructural support. It is lonely and isolating work. Some agencies have given us resources; many have denied us help. Others have, in my opinion, poached our ideas and/or taken credit for them. That is the story, unfortunately, told by many outsider voices in history.

However, patient leaders meet amazing people along the way – not just fellow travellers in the patient world, but also astonishing and generous spirits: nurses, physios and other health professionals who lend a hand to getting an idea implemented. Managers who glimpse the possibilities we bring and create the space. Admin staff who are incredible allies as they share an affinity with the problems we face – those on the psych ward, at the receptionist booth, who clean up the sick and wheel our tired bodies along long white corridors with walls of peeling paint.

And more and more, the work of patient leaders is recognised as being sorely needed, as the healthcare system lurches from one crisis to another and does not know, on the whole, how to 'do' partnership properly or work with us. I hope this book can help staff and institutions as well as budding patient leaders themselves.

Meanwhile, we also take inspiration from a wider patient and citizen movement that has at times needed to go it alone – that values independence and integrity, as well as yearning for true partnership. Only by rebalancing the scales by adding a weight to one side can you equalise power.

We know that patient leadership borrows from the history of community activism. We acknowledge the way that community development sees people bringing 'assets' to the table. We understand the rights-based movements pioneered by people with learning disabilities and mental health conditions, the maternity movement and HIV activists.

We stand on the shoulders of activists who have battled to improve safety after scandals such as thalidomide, from Bristol through Alder Hey and Winterbourne to Mid Staffs.

We have seen the emergence of a utilitarian patient movement focused on quality improvement in long-term conditions, such as cancer. The past few years have seen the rise of new forms of engagement that bolster the work, such as online dialogue, experience-based co-design, health champions, peer support and the like.

We admire those collective spirits pushing for more 'person-centred' care or shared decision-making. And we are fans of those who have always advocated for patient rights and statutory voice.

So many tributaries to the patient, community and citizens' movements in health! And, while we are at it, let's add the wider civil rights movements – feminism, LGBT, black and minority struggles, the ecologists and many more.

Patient leadership is one more tributary. In the current frenzied healthcare climate that loves its acronyms and shiny phrases – it is a true social movement. And it reaches around the world (hello to my friends in Canada at the Patient Advisory Network!).

What makes patient leadership unique is that it reframes illness as a gift – a painful gift, but nonetheless a gift. Yes, it is agonising and isolating and strips you of your identity. But it brings us closer to being human. And if we want to rehumanise our healthcare systems – to place what matters at the centre of our endeavour and rebuild relationships – then patient leaders must be part of solutions.

More broadly, the story of patient leadership also helps us see that the history of the healthcare system is an embattled one that takes place above the heads (and bodies and minds) of patients themselves.

In the UK, one can narrate the story of the NHS as a continuous battle to 'represent' the voices of patients by other institutional forces. Clinical (primarily medical) tribes proclaim to know what is best for us. Managerial and policy leaders likewise. Both 'own' our voices. It is time to speak for ourselves.

The journey and the magic

There are many books on autobiographical tales of suffering. There are many books by doctors whose perspectives have been transformed by being patients themselves. But little has been said by patients themselves about their wider work – beyond personal healing – undertaken 'professionally' and to which is brought passion, insight, expertise, humanity and a whole heap of other skills that have been undervalued in the past by leadership experts.

This book focuses on extraordinary patient leaders. This is not a scientific study. This is not a representative sample. This is not totally inclusive. Trigger warning: This book mentions suicide as well as drug and substance abuse.

This is the story of our 'gang' – those of us who had a dream that one day patient leaders and patient leadership would equalise power, that we would work alongside managerial and clinical leaders at local, regional, national and international levels, in policy making and across research, training and education, and service delivery.

As each chapter shows, the route towards being a patient leader is exciting, hard and dangerous (literally in some cases, as the effort often brings reward in the form of re-lapse). But it is also incredibly worthwhile.

This book is not about heroic victories. All those featured here have had an incredibly bumpy journey. Two steps forward, one step back – sometimes that step back feels like three, at least. Some have succeeded in doing what they set out to do. Others have diverted along the way. One or two have given up. Almost.

I am not going to do spoilers. But there are some themes that seem to crop up again and again during our struggles to equalise power.

Connection is critical. With ourselves, others and the world. Losing connection with – being at odds with – our previously balanced mind or healthy body is the epitome of pain and suffering. Losing connections with others while being ill can be devastating. And losing who we are in the world, equally so: who we were is not who we are; who we will be is not what we had hoped. Loss of meaning, purpose and identity are at the black heart of ill health.

And our deep understanding of the above is one reason why 'patients' value healing relationships, why they know so much about trust (and distrust), vulnerability and power, fairness and unfairness. Regaining connection is critical to healing. And a connected human health system is what we need. Who better to lead that movement than us? Those with skin in the game.

We also need to stop seeing 'patients' as only weak. The pain is real. But we are strong by dint of what we have had to face. This is not so much 'resilience' as moving through territories of immense danger. This is archetypal. In some senses people who have been affected by life-changing illness, injury or disability are the 'wounded heroes' of myth.

This knowledge is akin to shamans and wounded healers and visionaries. But our society has labelled 'illness' as weakness or a problem to be fixed. Thus, we have turned patients away from their 'personhood' and agency. The NHS then becomes blind to the value of us being equal partners in decision-making at all levels of the system.

Further, patient leaders going back into the fray to surface deeper meaning from their everyday heroism tell a tale of moving beyond 'ego' towards a collective strength and belief in wider humanity. 'One does not ask of one who suffers: What is your country and what is your religion? One merely says: You suffer, that is enough for me,' said Louis Pasteur in a speech to the Philanthropic Society in 1886.

That's a bit grandiose – read the chapters. You'll see what I mean!

The magic comes when the wisdom gained during suffering meets the wisdom that had been lost when one got ill in the first place (life experiences, capabilities, professional expertise). Everyone in this book has harnessed what they have learned during illness together with their 'previous' life skills to create something deeper – an enriched expertise. In order to help others. It is as if the heat of forged wisdom through suffering melts the 'frozen assets' and releases action in a new way.

And when the combined insights and passions of a patient leader connect with people in healthcare who are open, another magic starts to stir. Many times, it is the patient in the room who brings people back to their humanity, their vulnerability, perhaps the reason why they went into practising healthcare in the first place. To paraphrase Corporal Jones in *Dad's Army*, 'Permission to be human, sir.'

But the personal challenges of working with health professionals – how to balance being critical and creative, challenging and supportive; trying to foster partnerships from a position of powerlessness – are legion. You need strategies and tactics; you need to be able to influence, question, challenge assumptions and just keep going!

As Dominic Stenning sums up in his chapter, 'Can you put yourself out there in a healthy way?' Too many patient leaders crash and burn, or at least relapse. This is difficult work – managing your own energy, dealing with emotions, anger, the triggering of it all. Above all the isolation – those who succeed seem to have incredible support networks.

The process of writing the book has itself been fascinating. We have tried to work together – to 'model' the collaborative nature of our endeavour. For each chapter, I have sat down for a chat with my friends, recorded and then transcribed the recording. I then drafted a first chapter and sent it out and we collaborated on the second draft. Some made 'track changes'; some took control of the writing.

There were challenges to writing that mimicked much of the self-doubt we often have had. There were questions about how much people wanted to say and issues concerning disclosure. Several felt guilty about their stories not being 'interesting' or 'successful'. One or two of the 'gang' declined to be interviewed for their own good reasons. By the way, these are all personal opinions – the usual disclaimers apply!

We came together in January 2019 to discuss the book,

our own chapters and this introduction. And we have continued to share our writings. The launch event itself will be a celebration of how we can work together.

Since our Winchester origins, we have met many more times with the wider gang. We gossiped, moaned, celebrated, shared, even cried together. We had more than our healthy share of cake and planned, plotted and had more cake. And we supported each other on the journeys described in the following chapters. Ten years ago, the phrases 'patient leader' and 'patient leadership' did not exist. Our stories have been more and more visible since then.

And, while you read, please take a moment to remember Rosamund Snow (1971–2019). She was a friend, and much more. There is no doubt in my mind that there would have been a chapter here dedicated to her work, as academic, researcher, communication specialist, the first *British Medical Journal* Patient Editor, cat-lover, activist, colleague and mischief-maker.

We hope you will take the book as a gift for the next chapter of your own story.

There are one or two people to thank in particular (and many I have missed I am sure). Annie Laverty, Chief Experience Officer at Northumbria Healthcare NHS Foundation Trust, and Nick Goodman and his team at MES for their generosity – money to help write this book. The friendly editors and staff at Jessica Kingsley Publishers for their advice and encouragement – for taking a punt on me and not making too many changes to the copy. And those at Nesta for offering to host the launch!

To my very special mentor and friend Harry Cayton who

has been with me through many downs and more ups. And, of course, loads of fellow patient leaders, NHS staff and colleagues – too many to mention. But they are all part of trying to make sure the NHS focuses on what matters and heals.

This is the end of the beginning.

YOU HAVE TO BE THREE TIMES AS GOOD...

Michael Seres

You can get sexy knickers and sewage plumbing, but you can't get something to stop you shitting the bed at night. What if I could give the doctors the information they needed in real time? That's when my brain got going.

In October 2011, Michael woke up in a hospital bed, covered in shit. Literally.

A bowel transplant had saved his life and he was only the 11th person in the UK to receive one. His cares should have been over. But another phase of his life and career were just beginning.

'I had a bag attached to my body that was collecting my shit. It was overflowing and I couldn't do a thing about it.'

The surgeon and other health professionals told him this was normal and he should get used to it. But clinicians don't have to live with the consequences of a condition or treatment. It is the experience of the everyday that makes the patient leader a bit different: 'For the docs it was about survival, but the only thing I could think about was this bloody bag attached to my body.'

In hospital, they had to empty the bag and measure its contents. When he eventually went home he had to drain his shit from the bag into a bucket or big bag. He had to get extra sheets for his bed, obtain pastes and sachets to thicken the faeces so it did not leak. Companies were sending him special rucksacks for the bag, bedsheets, sprays, creams, barriers... 'My head was going, "This is just not normal, why does it need to be like that?" I was having conversations all the time about how much thickener to use.'

'The transplant was supposed to give me a quiet life.' His life since then has been anything but. He did his own research and, having a marketing and PR background, was determined to do something about it. He also describes himself as a 'pain in the arse' – unwilling to accept the status quo.

He used social media to connect with other patients to find out whether they were having similar problems. It was shocking to find others who suffered this sort of humiliation and discomfort in private: 'I connected with 20,000 patients. Everyone came back to me and said, "Yes, get used to it," or, "It's not that bad."'

He started questioning things – the default mode for a nascent patient leader: 'Why does it have to be that way?' And, fortunately, he had a surgeon who also became curious.

His first entry into the mindset of an entrepreneur though was triggered by his kids and a bout of boredom in hospital.

His family had just visited him on a Sunday afternoon: 'My kids had wheeled my IV [intravenous] trolley down to the cafe. And had been blowing up surgical gloves and sticking them on a pin board. I was thinking – why did everything to do with hospital care need to be so damn grey and boring? And these stoma bags? We can do better than this. Why can't you have your football team logo on it or a picture of your boss? You could shit on them. My daughter at that time was into Disney princesses – why can't we do that?'

Having a business background and being naturally curious, he looked into the options. 'Patients don't stop being people when they get ill.' Then he laughs: 'But I never thought we would be where we are.'

Michael had spent much of his career in consumer product licensing; in other words, building products and brands for other people. The licensing of *Who Wants to be a Millionaire?*, wooden toys with kids' favourite characters, t-shirts and apparel for football tournaments. Michael was always into building new products.

Now, the more serious task was dealing with overflowing faeces. Again, the idea came to him during the boredom and mundanity of dealing with the practical consequences of his lifesaving operation. He was at home, filling in spreadsheets for the doctors about what he had eaten, how much poo had come out and when and emailing them with the data. And by now the problems were not just overflow, but bacterial overgrowth, dehydration and infections.

For doctors and health professionals generally, these 'invisible' problems are not what matters. They may deal with the consequences, for example the readmissions and infections, but they don't see what matters to a person's daily life and they are not in a position to be able to prevent such things happening. And they don't deal in shit.

His first idea was to design a Bluetooth sensor alert to check on how fast the bag was filling up: 'We had to start somewhere. I believed that we could change the bag.' However, the implications of such a device were enormous. If you could change the way of measuring volume, you could also get better at automatic data collection. And, if you can link that to remote communication with hospitals and professionals, that could avoid readmissions to hospital for dehydration: 'What if I could give the doctors the information they needed in real time? That's when my brain got going.'

He was also seeing a private healthcare industry focusing on the wrong things. He had investigated other so-called 'innovative' solutions: 'The NHS will pay a company to plumb a tube from your bag into the sewage pipe so that shit can quietly drain away overnight.' He then mentions an inspirational entrepreneur who has designed lingerie for people with gut conditions: 'You can get sexy knickers and sewage plumbing, but you can't get something to stop you shitting the bed at night.'

At the same time, he was asked to give talks by his transplant team, partly to help identify and recruit other transplant patients, partly as medical education – this seems a common route in for patient leaders (see the chapters on Sibylle Erdmann and Alison Cameron). He had a credible understanding of the system due to his long-term problems. He also was able to provide advice on how to look after oneself through diet and nutrition, and this holistic approach gained credence amongst patients and staff alike. Meanwhile, Michael started blogging about his story and work. He has subsequently used social media to develop global online communities of thousands of patients. His blog has over 100,000 followers.

Michael's story is an illustration of how healthcare need is almost invariably defined through a professional and institutional lens. And thus there are significant blind spots, often to do with how one lives with a condition. Patients know what matters. But when they came up with solutions, they are easily ignored. Michael's struggles as an entrepreneur were only just beginning.

Having initially hacked a sensor by purchasing the product online and using video tutorials, Michael quickly realised that scaling a good idea was a massive challenge. He found manufacturing partners willing to build a product. One of his stand-out memories during this period was of 300 units being shipped to an exhibition in Florida. The box arrived and Michael eagerly opened it to find that the batteries had been left on and nothing worked. Now a battery 'pull tab' seems obvious.

Michael won some awards. Tech London Advocates awarded him 'new innovation of the year' and the Science Museum featured his device as part of a Patients as Innovators exhibition.

By now, Michael was starting to ask more fundamental questions: he wanted to know who made decisions about whether the NHS would pay for his product. This opened his eyes to the NHS and its opaque decision-making systems, codes and behaviours. And the huge barriers it puts up to innovation, particularly ideas that come from outside the system. He drew on his professional interest in legal and marketing issues to start shining a light on the fusty world of innovation, regulation and licensing. It wasn't a pretty sight.

'What became very clear very early on was that nobody was going to pay for my product in the UK.' He launches into the story of how he tried to get the NHS to support him in getting his product into the market and how it might be covered by the NHS. He discovered the 'drug tariff' – a list of treatments and procedures that the NHS would pay for. And he tried to get his product listed. Eighteen weary, bureaucratically inept months later, he was still trying: 'I saw all the other stuff they pay for, and thought, "Why not mine?"'

At first, there had been a Word document on a website to fill in. So he filled it in. Three months later, he got a note back saying, 'Where is your health economics model?' He then went back and said that the form had not asked for that and he didn't even know what a health economics model looked like. He went back and learned about that and hired some people to help him do one. They built the product, put it on 80 patients, looked at the benefits and delivered the findings – and of course he had to raise the finance for all this. They showed a 30% reduction in costs in terms of drug spend and reduced hospital admissions. He waited for the drug tariff team to get back to him. And waited. And waited. He heard nothing for another six months.

They finally replied and said they now needed a clinical evaluation. He had assumed that this was part of what he had already done. So, yet again, he went back and did what they had asked, bringing in his clinical team to help.

This demonstrated the benefits again and looked at how many people would use it and how it could be used in a clinical environment. And again it came from his own money. And another year went by.

Things were beginning to get on his nerves: 'They made it very clear that you can't talk to them; everything has to be done on email. This was bullshit. I was getting nowhere and being fobbed off.' Like most patient leaders entering the world of healthcare policy, he was up against systematic barriers to inclusion.

For many – particularly when it affects one's health (again) – this is the point at which people wave the white flag. Michael tried another tack. He challenged the tariff itself and questioned its relevance: 'I said, "I don't understand; you've got loads of stuff on the tariff." And no one would give me a straight answer.'

At this stage, Michael was relying on the generosity of an initial investor who believed in what he was doing. The investor, a pharmacist, understood the challenges Michael was trying to solve. It was his initial money that allowed him to take a handmade hack and turn it into a viable product. With that seed money he started to navigate the regulatory landscape and began to see the gulf between the UK and US systems. And he was about to get a dose of the UK system.

He was told there was a 'special way' in which products like this might go on what was then called an 'innovation tariff'. NHS England, an emerging quango at that stage, told him that his sort of product was 'exactly' what the system was looking for.

He was encouraged to apply for a new initiative called

'NHS Innovators' as an entrepreneur who would then get support. But again this was a dead end. He didn't get on to the programme. The goalposts shifted yet again. He was then told he didn't have to get on to this programme for his product to be regarded as ripe for the tariff. But his hopes were dashed once more, and his product was not listed on the new tariff after all.

'On the new list were episiotomy scissors, walk-in clinics and other stuff. I said, "What's going on?", and they said, "Sorry, we screwed it up. Could you help us rewrite the tariff? We'd love your input."' At this point in the interview, he leans back and rolls his eyes.

He was now experiencing another side of the patient leadership game – being asked to contribute his expertise for free: 'I gave them all the information about what we were doing and our experience in the US, as we had started production there. They sucked my brains. I was told to apply again last year and then got another rejection, as it did not fit with key priorities. I said fuck it and forget it.'

Other patient leaders, faced with such problems, have little energy left to make their mark. Or are so isolated and ill, they give up. Such talent wasted. This at a time when the NHS is desperate for new ideas.

I ask Michael about what he has learned: 'In the UK, all innovation is clinician driven, professionally driven; the role of the patient is not seen as useful. We are not valued in that way. The penny dropped only recently. Put aside for a moment that we are financially bankrupt; it is shambolic how we are trying to scale up technology. The system only trusts health professionals.'

He has all but given up on the UK. 'I can't be bothered any more. I spent £80,000 on clinical trials in eight places in the UK, knowing that patients won't be able to get it on the NHS.'

He refers to the complex architecture put in place recently in the health academic and research world – where new acronyms have to be learned, the world of AHSNs (Academic Health Science Networks), CLAHRCs (Collaborations for Leadership in Applied Health Research and Care) and NHS innovation and so-called entrepreneurs. 'They are stuffed full of "clinical champions". But there are no "patient entrepreneurs".'

He apologises: 'Sorry for getting too passionate. It is fine for me because I now have my own company and I am ballsy. I will get the meetings with high-up folk – I will share the story – but I will not be able to scale something up because I am not clinical. This is a perfect example of the old world colliding with the new world.'

Michael founded 11 Health (11 is a special number, because of Michael being the 11th person in the UK to have bowel transplant surgery). And he has had to leave this country in order to succeed. He turned to the US for funding after being turned down in the UK 43 times. He found a US investor – 'a legend in Silicon Valley' – who has subsequently become his mentor and friend. 'That initial money came with two caveats: 1. Don't run your company like a British company; 2. You have to move to the US.'

That is exactly what Michael did. Starting with one desk in a co-working space, Michael has now built a team of 35 based in Southern California. He has turned the original sensor into the world's first smart care platform for stoma patients, which includes the first ever smart bag.

'Now technology can help manage the shit and we can learn from what comes out of the body and exactly what to put back in. The company doesn't see distribution of its product as something that should be any different to other consumer items. We will ship your medical supplies in the same way as anything else.'

At a strategic level: 'My job is simple. Surround myself with brilliant people who are far cleverer than me and steer the ship.'

However, this is not just about technology. Michael's greatest passions have always been helping others and how patients can help other patients. This has been boosted by his own experiences, where family and friends were the sole support – 'the unsung heroes' – and another 'care gap'. He noted that patients as peer support workers are a hugely undervalued resource.

At 11 Health, they coach patients to buddy other patients and measure the outcomes.

He has utilised his understanding around peer support to found a business model for delivery of his products: 'We have changed the way we deliver the service. We have 15 patient champions who have stomas, who have not been able to get back to work. They can work for us, for an hour, part time or full time. They go into a hospital and they link up with other patients, not to sell the product, but to see if they can help. The app we produce is full of educational resources.'

It is not a patient takeover. This is collaborative work.

The doctors are engaged too: 'We have doctors phoning us up to ask for help and to find a patient they can bring in to talk to their own patients about how to live post-operatively with a transplant.'

Meanwhile, Michael has harsh words for what happens in the UK. While he is treated almost like a celebrity when he walks on to a national event stage, nothing has changed behind the scenes. 'The NHS continues to spout its empty rhetoric about "patients being at the centre" and about being at the forefront of innovation.'

'I started looking at all the research and innovation coming through and there was another app announced recently about waiting times... They are all clinician driven, all insider driven, and I have this naive belief about patient centricity.' He pauses: 'It's bullshit. It may be kicking off in terms of a few old-fashioned patient groups in GP surgeries or low-level engagement in hospitals, but there is no real power in the system.'

He mentions the role I have currently, as a patient director. In fact, Michael was the first person I met who had the idea of patients as chief executives. 'Nobody is acting on it. There should be a patient CEO in every healthcare organisation. Until that happens, this movement cannot flourish. Everybody goes, "Yes, lovely idea," and then nobody does anything.'

As someone who has had mental health problems and is interested in the emotional effects of physical health problems, I ask him about how he keeps his mind healthy. 'There is zero understanding of mental effects of long-term physical health problems. If you have trauma, there will be inevitable one-off mental health issues to deal with. But if you are living with chronic complex conditions where there is no chance of "getting better", that is a huge psychological consequence and it never gets addressed. Everyone repeats, "Are you OK?", but nothing follows... My mind and gut are totally related but they are never treated together.'

Once again, he points out the love and support he has had: 'I am lucky I have family and work as therapy and my escape. I look at those who do not have those other outlets or those who choose not to have those outlets; I see cases spiralling out of control.'

This is not just a personal issue; it also has huge implications for the prevention and integration agenda. He tells me about people who have had transplants coming in again because they have not been able to deal with the problems that led to them needing a transplant the first time. 'There are two patients in hospital, one on kidney and bowel transplant, none of their issues have been addressed – drug abuse, unstable home environment, living conditions.' Once again, it is patients who see the impact of siloed working at first hand, can point out its effects, could help come up with solutions.

Michael seems to have become a bit of a celebrity in some circles, often giving international presentations and being invited onto expert committees; he is a published author and a professional speaker. He is the inaugural e-patient in residence and an executive board member at Stanford Medicine X. He has helped implement the first Skype clinics in the Oxford University Hospitals Trust and is an ambassador to the prestigious Doctors 2.0 conference.

But his feet remain firmly grounded. And he still speaks truth to power. 'For all the US health system dysfunction, they have recognised our innovations. In the UK, it is all about who holds power.'

'We [patients] have as many qualifications, as much knowledge, as many professional qualities, just a different set of skills; for healthcare to move forward properly, everyone has to have a seat around the table, at equal level.'

He qualifies this slightly: 'I don't want to be around the table because I am "just" a patient; it is because I am also Michael Seres. I want them to say, "He also runs a business, understands strategy and budgeting, can contribute in the same way."'

In other words, how he sees things is different but equal, like all others in this book. We are no better and no worse than a surgeon or a nurse, a financial manager or an IT worker. But the value must be equal. As he puts it, 'I am not fighting for "us" above them, only for a level playing field.'

He sees a few, but not many, similar entrepreneurs and is pained by their struggles – he mentions Denise Stephens, founder of Enabled by Design, in particular as a 'hero'. But he sees few examples of patient-led companies, though he makes an exception for PatientsLikeMe – a space for online patient groups that was set up in response to the personal experiences of its founder.

Unsurprisingly, he already has eyes on the next step: 'If I have the time and the money, we could bring together a patient resource. I want a patient CEO in every healthcare organisation. And I want my company to start an incubator for patients as entrepreneurs.'

I delve backwards as well as forwards. What in his background has made him the way he is? He was diagnosed with the incurable bowel condition, Crohn's disease, at the age of 12. It was only following over 20 operations and an intestinal failure that he had the transplant. Michael has also been a cancer patient (twice) due to his lowered immune system, a result of drug side effects.

'My healthcare journey is relatively unremarkable, because every one of us has a story.' I am well versed in Michael's humility. We have been friends for a long time now.

His diagnosis of Crohn's disease followed two years of being told he was faking his stomach aches: 'An irony, because I wanted to go to school. I was good at sports; it was all I wanted to do. I was one of the youngest cricket captains they had, played for Middlesex schools, captain of Camden schools, rugby scrum half.'

Back then Crohn's disease was a rare thing; now, IBD (irritable bowel disease) is well known. It was often treated with high-dose steroids. Not pretty for a kid. He was a 'geeky, awkward teen', but now had to deal with a bloated face, rashes and extra bad moods. He needed surgery at 14, and when he came back to his school in north London, he had his first real taste of discrimination. Why was the seat next to him at assembly left empty? It seemed the staff felt his disease was contagious.

Do patient leaders have an inbuilt sense of the unfairness and injustice of life? Is it intertwined with their personality or their journey? Their family life or their healthcare experience? 'I always had a mouth on me but I was basically a good kid – compliant.' But that critical mind was there from the off: 'I could challenge and question and found my voice on the cricket field.'

His teen years were littered with health problems: 'They knew me at the Royal Free. "What are you here for this time?" the receptionist would ask. I was the one who emerged from the scrum with a broken wrist... I didn't know then that Crohn's could affect bone density. We always thought it was sporting accidents. I was diagnosed with ankylosing spondylitis, was in a lot of discomfort – it became a joke. I spent a year on crutches with ligament pain.'

Frustrated by his school's attitude and losing out on learning through his breaks in hospital, he went to a tutorial college, Albany College, to make up for his missed O levels. And there he found the sort of support, enthusiasm and encouragement that had been missing from his schooling thus far.

Michael is big on support. He weaves that message through everything he says. And Albany College offered him everything he needed to take his frustrated, opinionated, curious mind that step further. 'The amazing English teacher came to teach me at the bedside in hospital.'

But that didn't mean he agreed with anyone. 'I loved the debate, the intellectual jousting, and of course, because of what I had been through, I wasn't always willing to back down... I had two brilliant teachers for law and politics who left their mark – in the case of politics, their left-wing mark! I always took the opposite view. I also enjoyed the case law; health was always a big thing – we talked about the NHS, constitutional and social welfare stuff. I was fascinated by inequalities.'

He also had an eye for business that would help later on. His family was in the 'schmutter business'. His father, a second-generation East End Jew with Russian roots, was a clothing manufacturer and Michael spent his summers helping out at a bristle factory owned by his grandfather on his mum's side. 'Only a handful of my grandparents' family survived the holocaust.' He pauses. 'Summer was great. It was time with grandpa, with dad. I enjoyed the business background on both sides of the family – going to the factory. It always led to Blooms [the famous Jewish salt-beef sandwich makers]. I remember the buildings and people vividly. One aunt was a designer, the other did the books; it was a real family business – loved it.'

So, perhaps he had talents to fall back on? Perhaps his curious mind and professional interests made him ripe to re-enter the healthcare world with a whizz. He certainly had the support, which is crucial for most of us. Even so, what he did was and is remarkable.

Like me, he was a good sportsman at school. Like me, he supports a rubbish football team with a decent pedigree: 'My cousin took me to see Queens Park Rangers at Loftus Road in the early 1970s when I was six and we lost to Liverpool in the league by a point. I am still waiting to see us win a trophy.' Maybe our frustration comes out in our work!

Having listened to his story for a couple of hours, I ask him the question that haunts me: why bother? 'Because we care and because it's not right, and I think we do it because there is a bit of activism in us, I think we all have a commonality to different levels, a feistiness, a cause, a belief in trying to right an injustice in a way.'

He has a final thought: 'Patient leaders have to deal with their own conditions, they have to be extra good to break into and change the system and they have to be as good a leader as those who are in the system – we need to be three times as good as those who have been brought up culturally entitled to a leadership position. We have to be three times as good to be treated as an equal.'

MAKING THE CONNECTION

Kate James

It's that deeper, human connection that makes the world go round. Relationships are fundamental. The beauty in patient leaders delivering this work is the humanity in it – that's what makes it successful, that's what makes it so difficult. That's what makes it so heart-breaking and so unbelievably rewarding.

Kate has been looking after others since she was a kid. Though she says she finds it difficult to see herself as a patient leader, she has been trying to make things better for fellow patients, carers and staff since she was ten.

She was five when she had a tonsillectomy and ten when she was diagnosed with diabetes (later discovered to be as a result of a split pancreas that led to pancreatitis), and Ward 25 at the Luton and Dunstable Hospital became her home from home during the 1990s: 'I grew up on a children's ward.'

She was often admitted with ketoacidosis (excessive blood sugar levels): 'Mum would call them and say I needed to come in. There was an enormous sense of familiarity and security in that.'

It is easy for an outsider to see that many of the qualities that she possesses and uses in her work were forged back then. First, her sense of self-responsibility and independence, self-leadership if you like. Her parents encouraged her to take control of her illness: 'They said, "This is your diabetes, take responsibility," which I did, gladly.' 'In fact,' she laughs, 'I never let anyone else near me with injections and things like that.'

Her natural, scientific curiosity – always trying to puzzle things out and wanting to learn – led her to asking a lot of questions: 'I wanted to know about what was going on, more than my own care. I would read the little clipboard at the end of the bed, fascinated. I was always asking questions, even when I was unwell. I was a sickly child and needed to understand what was going on with me and my body.'

She talks about 'fond memories' of hospital – of a nurse who would chat to her for ages and a friend who would chat late at night. Of a student nurse regaling her with questions for an assignment on her experiences. 'I chatted to her for hours. I wanted everyone to know that I could look after myself. At ten, I knew it was either that or become too dependent on others.'

Her sense of independence sometimes morphs into a clear recognition of her own latent mischievousness – itself rooted in childhood ('I would run off with my brother, climb trees, get injured'). She also likes to have fun and is still a risk taker (I got to know Kate at about the time she did a sponsored charity skydive).

She invokes another hospital memory: 'I fancied this boy who'd broken his leg. When I went home at the weekend, I would bring him back goodies, like Coke and Mars Bars. We did have fun – unhooking curtain rails, watching films together, dancing on the tables in the schoolroom, skating down the corridors on drip stands.'

She pauses. 'It wasn't a holiday camp though, surely?' I ask. She nods. 'Maybe part of those memories and tales of fun come from wanting to protect my family – those closest to me – from the reality of what I was living through. Even things like not being able to go to the toilet because I was attached to tubes, not being able to get dressed as I was wired up. No dignity. No privacy. Painful interventions like getting blood gases done. The sounds from the treatment room of children screaming... But I didn't want my family to know how awful that was, and those nights alone when you are just crying silently, because you are so lonely and so scared.'

The sense of caring for others was instilled in her at an early age: 'For reasons I do not yet fully understand, I was the mother figure child, making sure the younger ones were OK.' She tells of a three-year-old called Sam, who was in for appendicitis. She later became friends with him and his family.

That sense of continuity and community is precious. And extends to staff. 'Even at that age, I was very aware of the underlying tensions with staff and systems, processes that got in the way of care. I remember being acutely aware that staff were stressed.'

Like many patients and service users, she found herself looking after others to protect them from their own anxieties. She certainly wanted 'to make sure everyone else was OK'. Kate is still trying to find the boundaries that help her work, live and protect herself. The roots are to be found in the fact that both her grandads died when she was young and her dad when she was 31. But, 'It was not something we talked about.' Full stop.

As any cod psychologist like me knows, these protective devices don't always wear well in the long term. Our defensive mechanisms can be strengths and later weaknesses. For people with long-term health conditions, or those who go into trying to change the system, they can come back to bite. She agrees, to a certain extent: 'Lately I have come to realise it is also not necessarily the best way to look after yourself.' It is interesting to note that when I meet Kate for the book, she is in the process of making radical changes to her life, partly based on a recent bout of work-related stress.

Back then as an adolescent, she wanted to study medicine, unsurprisingly. Though that dream was not realised, the work she does now feeds her fascination with health, medicine and science. She is more than comfortable within healthcare settings and with health professionals, which has enabled her to thrive in medical environments.

Having seen her deal with all sorts of staff (managerial, admin, clinical) and patients in the work we now do together, I see where this all comes from. Since patient leadership is all about building trusting relationships in order to influence decision-making, this stands her in good stead: 'It doesn't faze me, whether I am chatting to someone serving the coffee or the CEO.'

Having had pretty horrible experiences on a psychiatric ward, I find this difference in attitude intriguing. She builds on my thought: 'People who have been in hospital, either never want to set foot in the place again or they do want to be part of it. I still get a kick out of being in that environment, I really enjoy it. I am confident and comfortable, especially in busy teaching hospitals.'

Being a bit of a melancholic soul, I push on with this part of the discussion. She agrees that hospitals are places of illness, pain and suffering. But she holds on to an almost feverish sense of hope, which I find compelling: 'Part of it is because of my knowledge of what's going on – yes, all the terrible stuff, utter despair, death and heartache, but also the development, progress, research and all of that. Hope. That's what is exciting.'

Her dream of doing medicine withered during her teens, partly because of plummeting self-confidence that edged into mental health problems. Come her GCSE exams, she was in many ways in deep distress beneath outward appearances. She felt awkward socially, began to miss school and then changed schools mid-term one year. Capturing some sense of identity within the whirlwind of ill health, common to many patient leaders, was a looming problem: 'At the new school, I was the new person but did not know who this person was.'

Her first overdose was at 16. Recognition as to why came later – that loss of identity, fear of failure and subsequent dream-breaking acknowledgement that she wouldn't go into medicine.

'Looking back, I was very depressed. It manifested in more physical ways – stomach or back aches.'

I have often been curious about suicide and am struck by the hard-nosed way in which she describes that first overdose: 'I made the decision that I would see in the new year, then on the third of January I took loads of paracetamol and did not expect to wake up to take my exams.'

And then I am equally shocked by her casual description of what happened next. Because she had been so unwell previously and was physically sick a lot, the overdose went unnoticed. Kate did not tell anyone (there is that self-reliance gone too far) and managed to hide it from everyone. Fortunately, her liver and kidneys were undamaged; ironically, perhaps due to the fact that, because of pancreatitis, the toxic chemicals were not fully absorbed. She dubs all this a 'terrible resilience' due to a need to protect others.

And from one extreme to another, she got on 'as if nothing happened' and went on the best holiday of her life a few weeks later – a ten-day skiing trip to Denver where she felt exhilarated by a sense of achievement on the slopes: 'I am capable of enjoying stuff as well as being capable of deep, utter desperation, somehow to get out of that box and enjoy the moment, as if living two parallel lives.'

For the first time, she felt a sense of freedom and perspective, a refreshing sense of 'normality' and a fresh lease of life – even a romance! She passed her GCSEs, albeit still in 'physical turmoil' with her pancreatitis. Page after page of her diaries described total exhaustion and a desire to sleep.

There is still a sense of wonderment in her voice that she is still alive. The struggle has continued until now. She is 40 and on the threshold of exciting opportunities; this is more my narrative than hers. Though she is gradually learning about real hope, I am also hoping – that these words get through to her when she reads them! 'At 16, I could not envisage a future, but now...' Her voice trails off. She is getting there.

Kate tends to underplay what she did in her 20s and 30s. But I see it as relevant. From a job helping people with mental health problems back into work ('co-production, though we did not then call it that') through working in a pharmacy ('I loved learning about medicines and helping customers') and then working in the charity sector, the real Kate was always popping up – independent, curious and caring.

But a second blow – deteriorating eyesight and loss of sight in one eye – prevented her from pursuing the second dream of studying pharmacy: 'I guessed I would not have been much good at dispensing methadone. Seriously, it was terrifying. Asking Mum whether I had my eyes open or not. And there I was learning about healthcare the hard way again.'

She describes herself as 'bouncing back somehow'. 'How?' I ask. 'I honestly don't know, so many things have happened. But always somehow, somewhere within me, even at my most depressed, I would get on with it.'

Kate remembers talking to secondary mental health staff about the employment project and someone commenting on her passion. 'I want people to be enabled to make decisions for themselves. There is such value in that – of having that person with different experiences and different perspectives able to look at things differently.' And yet, during this period working on the employment scheme, she tried to kill herself again.

And yet and yet: 'All the time, I wanted to ensure that the individual voice – not just mine – was heard within the healthcare system.' Contradictions or – better – inter-weavings, the personal and the professional bleeding into one another.

One of the main challenges remains – one we encounter again and again in the book: how she can maintain the permeability of mind and heart so as to help others and at the same time protect herself. Her recent job reminds her of this – working closely with people who are very ill and supporting them to understand their experiences reminds her deeply of her own experiences, distress and mortality.

We begin a discussion about the 'toolbox' that can help patient leaders look after themselves. She feels she is just beginning to build it for herself.

In many ways, Kate and I are mirror opposites. I need to stop 'leaking' my feelings, whereas she says she has always 'filtered' what she gives out about herself (though that does not affect what she lets in!). But her 'dam has burst recently'.

She is at an emotional crossroads and feels she has not 'processed' her own experience in a way that is 'helpful to me and for others'. Kate is nothing if not hard on herself and how far she has come. 'I feel that the personal and professional experiences or skills I have – the dedication, vision, passion – I can see in others. That is brilliant. But recently, the ability to identify with others who are very ill, I have found overwhelming. That makes me think I have bounced from one experience to another without processing it. That, plus being too young and busy.'

'Recently, I have seen such vulnerability, such incredible

bonds – people being able to be honest about what they have been through, what they have lost, what they have grieved for. That vulnerability, combined with the unfairness of it...', and here she tears up. 'What I have realised is the unfairness of what happened to me as a kid. It was really unfair that I had to go through all of that.'

She continues: 'I never allowed myself the thought "Why me?", but in the recent work there was an incredible amount of life brimming over in a room full of people that were dying, or living with the fear of dying, or going through horrendous physical painful treatments, intrusive and soul-destroying.' It was a combination of all these things that led to her latest phase of deep realisation that she needed time to pause and reflect – less of a bounce, more of a rest and a rebuilding.

And here we turn towards what's wrong with the healthcare system. The way it cannot flex to allow people (whether staff or patients) to process their experiences, reflect, learn and improve. 'You just have to get on with it, serving the client base, measurement and monitoring, funding pressures, the need for constant change and so-called innovation. That clash. That friction between the wellbeing of those you support and the need to deliver. Targets and paperwork, jumping through hoops. That constant fight.'

We pause. Then we find ourselves delving deeper. If this book is about healing the healthcare system via patient leadership, then what do we bring, as patient leaders, to help – to slow things down, to allow for deep change, to restore humanity? Whatever one feels the change needs to be. If we can't pinpoint that, then we are stuck and this movement is not worth the candle.

'It's that deeper, human connection that makes the world go round. Relationships are fundamental. The beauty in patient leaders delivering this work is the humanity in it – that's what makes it successful, that's what makes it so difficult. That's what makes it so heart-breaking and so unbelievably rewarding.'

And where does that deeper connection come from? Kate does not like the term 'suffering', and she feels 'living with' underplays the heart. 'Maybe it's about a shared understanding of an unwritten suffering. The boundaries can come down when a "patient" shares with a "patient" – it is an acknowledgement of that pain between two people without the boundaries. The healing comes from the sharing.'

'It sounds dangerously like love,' I joke. She says it's more about 'the bond of pain'. And at the same time, we say, 'Or both.'

'Yes. There is something so overwhelmingly positive about that human connection. Contrast that with what I can get from the majority of professionals. And the healthcare system as a whole – its systems and its processes. This inane focus on boundaries. It is, ironically, the professionalism that gets in the way of that connection. It is the breaking down of those boundaries that contains many of the answers.'

But professionals can be kind and compassionate too, I challenge. And loads of them have life-changing illness, injury or disability. What's the difference? 'Patient to patient – that hug would be almost the first thing you do. You don't have to think about it. It is a natural human reaction. You don't have to consider professional boundaries in the way that a medical professional does.'

I try to summarise this last part of the conversation. There seem to be two aspects of thinking about equal relationships between professionals (staff and leaders) and patients (individuals and patient leaders). One is about recognising what each brings in terms of understanding, knowledge or expertise. Another is what we have just been talking about – the need for a human connection, one more commonly found patient to patient – a 'connection through shared pain'. One is about the head and one the heart.

So, we should all cry together, I tease. 'No. Though I know now that if I put up too much of a boundary, that takes away from what I am able to do. I also know – or am trying to learn – that there must be ways to cope in that state of deep connection. Though I am still trying to find out how,' she laughs. I am sure she will discover it.

On a more practical level, Kate knows she has much to offer but feels scared of the consequences of being so vulnerable and open about her experiences. Like many of us, she is worried about being labelled as 'weak' or 'unreliable' in the job market. Her mantra is partnership. She highly respects the healthcare profession and the knowledge that individuals bring to the table. Her fears and frustrations lie in the hit-and-miss nature of that respect being returned.

However, the case for patient leaders is that life-changing illness, injury or disability has to be valued as an asset at the same time that suffering is acknowledged. Kate needs to earn a living, but it is a particularly difficult time to be doing this work: 'The system is so broken that it is a fragile place to be. This work can be unrecognised, yet needs to be done so urgently. I want to help make a system that has been so much part of me better. And I want to work with others to do that.'

One way through is by using art. Kate is working with me on using poetry and creative writing as a tool to bring people together in a safe environment, where all the traditional professional boundaries are removed. 'Art can do that. You are a group of human beings, you suffer and have pain, so the beauty is where you have respect for each other regardless of title and role. You value what each brings; that's when the magic happens.'

Through her years of experience of using and working within a healthcare setting, Kate has seen the good, bad and ugly when it comes to practice. She has been able to influence service redesign and inform research studies and is currently working with nursing students to ensure they have an insight into the patient experience in order to be the best future nurses. 'As patients, we have such a deep insight into what is missing. The simple things that can make a big difference. When you strip away process, procedure, paperwork – what matters most.'

And this brings us back to the reframing of patients as 'creatives' and 'healers' and the need to value our strengths rather than define us solely by our suffering: 'Actually I've handled more shit than most people could ever go through and I'm stronger because of it. I have managed my own health 24/7 for 30 years. I make hundreds of decisions a day to keep myself alive. I multitask and problem solve all day, every day. And that's before I've left the house! Yes, I am fragile. I have cracks right through my very soul, but as the saying goes – it's those cracks that let in the light.'

JEDI MASTER OF INVOLVEMENT

Dominic Stenning

Yes! We have changed things. There are times when we can all feel, 'Oh bloody hell, they're not listening,' but I do feel we've had a big impact on everything. It is also about a feeling of belonging – to be part of a kind tribe.

Over a Coke at lunchtime in a pub by a roundabout near Slough, Dominic professes that he is not so interested in his own story. Which is a bit of a pity, I think, because his story – particularly given our setting – is so extraordinary. But he insists: 'I want to talk about the work I am doing and how it affects me, draw on specific experiences. The story is valuable but I am sick of giving my story away for nothing. People don't link the experience with the expertise. I am more than the sum of what has happened to me.'

It seems a bold and justifiable stance. But this story is

not for nothing. It is worth sharing. Maybe it could change a lot of things...

'When my dad died, just after his 50th birthday, heroin filled the hole of grief remarkably well. I ended up injecting and drinking heavily for a long time.' Dominic went through various periods at rehab clinics but none worked: 'They're hopeless, as you are put in a false environment.' Once, he was put on barbiturates as part of a five-day radical detox so as to sleep through withdrawal effects. But this had severe bone pain and psychological consequences. 'It was unimaginably awful. For example, I hallucinated about my mate's dead dog being next to me in bed.'

On the way back from that detox... 'I just wanted to die 'cos all of a sudden I had these raw emotions I hadn't been feeling for the last decade. Like someone had torn the plaster off and I was suddenly exposed, and it was painful, plus all the things that had happened during those years, pretty nasty things. I was reliving all of that and I tried jumping out of the car. On the motorway – but try opening your door at 70mph with wind resistance!'

Dominic got off drugs by himself. 'To get clean, I had to cut off from everyone, lose old mates. I use the term "mates" loosely, though a lot of them really were, and I've lost many who've died. Every time I said I was going to get clean, I meant it. It is not manipulative. The final straw was when I was living in the tool shed at my gran's place. I was searching for a stash and was withdrawing. I realised Mum had had it with me. And that I'd had it too. That was the moment things changed.'

He got jobs in bars to keep his mind off the cravings.

He was on course for a solid rebuilding of his life and then chapter two of the story unfolded.

Just before Christmas in 2008, he wrecked his lumbar spine in a car accident. 'All that effort coming off drugs for what?' He ended up incapacitated in bed and was told he would kill himself within a year due to his ballooning weight – 33 stone and rising – and because of his lapse into drinking. He got through a litre of Jack Daniels most nights.

'You'd hear the bin men emptying ours of a ton of bottles. Mum would be looking at me. I put her through hell. But she stuck by me. I would not be here otherwise. When you are 33-plus stone, cannot move around the house and can barely use the toilet properly, you don't really want to live. I didn't have a future.'

The turning point was being offered a gastric bypass in 2011. Dominic rediscovered his immense and latent willpower. He realised this was another chance at life, lost four stone and stopped drinking preceding the operation to demonstrate his commitment. He also found himself a good therapist and, as he put it, 'life swung around'.

Ironically, the mental health team had been against the operation and had warned the local surgical team that it wasn't worthwhile because of Dominic's 'addictive' personality – this memory and stereotypes about the way drug users behave still rankle. And he also has strong views about the disconnection between mental health and drug services. But he prefers not to dwell on the past or hold lingering resentments. It is learning fodder.

Then, a few months after the operation, an occupational therapist who had stayed close asked Dominic to be on the steering group for the local recovery college – an emerging educational initiative to support people with mental health problems in rebuilding their lives.

Dominic was proud to be involved, as it played to his passion about co-production and working as equals. Was he perhaps too passionate? He laughs: 'Even then I wanted student representation on designing and delivering the programme. Ethics from the ground up. I was quite intense at the time. Maybe with the experience I have gained now, I might have resolved it, but I came up against a lot of opposition. I didn't take it very well.'

I ask him why he felt so strongly about the issue of student representation. Where did that drive for equity stem from?

'People say to me, "Oh you want to give back." They're kind of right, but I struggle with that 'cos it kind of implies that I am giving back from a debt I owe. I do it more for the reason that I want things to be better than what they were when I went through it. There were some good people in my care teams, but I have had really bad ones and the system has a thing about addicts and mental health service users, that they are manipulative and all sorts.'

Dominic pushed for more meaningful involvement at the recovery college and was reading avidly about co-production, hungry for the chance to engage with education again – to get the college to do more than getting feedback via questionnaires. 'Things needed to change and I really liked the ethos of the recovery college. But I wanted to hold their feet to the fire, to drive through the principles at all levels. If you say you're going to do that, then do it properly.'

I have always sensed Dominic's eager, curiosity-laden,

expansive intelligence. 'I like to be stimulated; this gave me a bit more oomph, but at the time I was argumentative.'

This tension between 'challenge' and 'support' crops up in many of the chapters in this book: 'I may not have helped my case. I felt pushed out, that the doors had shut on me 'cos I was too difficult.' And thus the circle of a patient leader's life may get played out: 'Then I get the rejection which is so familiar. Triggering. Like what happened in previous times of my life.'

I get a sense of affinity. Dominic, like many of us, wears his heart on his sleeve big time. And he can suffer for it. He is extremely open and insightful about his character. 'Because of what I have been through – the drugs, the drink, the sort of people I hung out with I suppose – I am generous but have been used, so am wary and hyper-vigilant.' I suggest that over-generosity and being used are common traits for patient leaders. He nods.

'Yeah. I wonder what keeps us going, putting our hand in the fire, again and again.' I am not sure I have an answer for this. Instead, I compliment him on his insight. But this is awkward for him too: 'I struggle with compliments. I've been through a lot and put others through it too. Mum lost my dad. My brother left and got married. In that time I tried to support Mum as best I could, but I was often scoring.'

This time I compliment him for his resilience and his humour – on the twinkle in his eye, the ability perhaps to laugh instead of cry. 'That'll be the "lack-of-respect-for-authority" twinkle,' he replies. 'More seriously – it is bloody hard, like learning when to say no, how to pick yourself up again, but I suppose we patient leaders are pretty practised at that.'

For a while, we dwell deeper in the past. Dominic was the son of a local GP and dropped out of school at 14, partly because of the bully of a headmaster. He often felt trapped as a child and was a 'bit of a nightmare' as a youngster. While under the care of a CAMHS (children and adolescent mental health services) team, he pinched his sister's car and drove 45 miles to Leicester.

When the psychiatrist lectured him, Dominic realised what he was doing – testing whether he could stand up to it. 'But then he told me to stop analysing him.' This mixture of acute insight and need to stand up to unfairness has stuck with him. For better and worse. A black belt in Taekwondo as an adolescent helped his sense of courage and brought him a sense of belonging and much-needed confidence as he grew up, before he turned to drugs when his father died.

We come back to his patient leadership 'career'. He is an outspoken advocate for the notion of 'patients as leaders', more vocal about it than many. He threw himself into the patient leadership programme, run by the Centre for Patient Leadership. This focused on developing the capabilities to be able to work in equal partnership with professional healthcare leaders. It had come at just the right time: 'I was thinking about what it is to be a leader, about integrity particularly. That's the strongest one for me, the foundation of everything. About courage and perseverance. I really got into it. I learned loads about listening actively instead of waiting to get your point in. I felt there was a lot more to this and got into learning about lots of other different types of leadership.'

But there was a deeper reason for his appetite: 'I had lost

my identity, 'cos I wasn't the Dominic before drugs, so who the fuck am I? This feeling of not knowing who I am, not having friends, being isolated. That is really tough. I had lost who I wanted to be and who I had been.'

Like Karen Owen, Alison Cameron and me, he gradually got into Twitter, and he set up a blog site and dubbed himself 'patient leader' on social media. For someone who had been, as he classed it, 'terrified' of going on Twitter at first, this strikes me as a bold pseudonym. 'After realising that I could expand on the blog, which was about letting people know how I was coping, I met people, and started learning more about healthcare – all those bloody acronyms, LTC, CCG... – and seeing what others were doing was fascinating and critical.'

But calling yourself a 'patient leader' in those days strikes me as a very Dominic thing to do – to strike out, while still admitting vulnerability: 'I thought I'd get a lot of shit for that, but fuck it. Someone said it seemed a very grandiose thing to do. Then Alison [Alison Cameron, who is a close friend] told the other guy, "You're just jealous that we have the audacity to come out and say it!" I thought, "Damn right." I really got behind that idea of patient leadership.'

Dominic pauses. As ever, he is thinking carefully about what he has just said. 'Alison summed it up brilliantly. As Brits we think, "Oh you can't call yourself a leader. You've got to play it down." But there's a bit of hidden snobbery here. If you're in a paid position, you get that bestowed upon you. It almost comes with the territory. We have to claim it for ourselves.'

He also sees the term as deliberately provocative. It

makes people sit up and question the term and perhaps think more deeply about the language we use: 'I wanted people to ask about patient leadership, so I thought I would make people sit up and challenge their thinking, and they'd come to ask me about it. It's a bit like sticking two fingers up. The term itself is in your face: "We may be patients, but we can be leaders like you." It challenges people's preconceptions; that's what I love about it.'

While he is talking, I think about how the gay community has reclaimed the words 'queer' and 'dyke'. How users of mental health services have reclaimed the word 'bonkers'. Words have meanings and stories behind them. And narratives can be retold.

Dominic continues: 'But I could really see how it could work. It has turned out to be more evolution than revolution. But I thought, and still think, this is going to get people to change things.'

'Have things changed?' I ask (slightly gloomily perhaps). 'Yes! We have changed things. There are times when we can all feel, "Oh bloody hell, they're not listening," but I do feel we've had a big impact on everything. It is also about a feeling of belonging – to be part of a kind tribe.'

And then came the break into national-level work. He was asked to be one of nine members of a service-user/patient (or what is now often called 'people with lived experience') panel on the Barker Commission – the independent Commission on the Future of Health and Social Care in England.

Once again, this was both exciting and tough. Dominic worked well with the convenor and project manager, Becky Seale. He came to be, he felt, the one to speak up for the group, particularly when the process was off-kilter. Knowing that Becky was under pressure too, there was a close affinity. He also ended up feeling a bit stuck in the middle and saw the challenges of stepping up – but he has never shied away from that.

At this time, as his blog kicked off and was well received, he was also starting to enjoy the glitz of conference opportunities. Like many patient leaders he was 'wheeled on' to tell his story and met influential professional leaders and once, memorably, was asked for a private, slightly surreal and impromptu discussion with the then Health Secretary Jeremy Hunt.

Meanwhile, there was also the inevitable backlash amongst established 'lay representatives' who had sat on worthy committees for years and perhaps felt this new wave of 'patient leadership' was a threat.

Maybe this comes with the territory for any leader who steps up? 'I have witnessed that jealousy. But if nobody takes the lead, I will. Then things get tense; others see me as taking over. But I just want to keep things going. I set the bar high for co-production.'

But the emotional kickback arrived as well: without support, he ran out of energy. About a year after the Barker Commission, he got asked to talk at a high-profile event. The pressure was becoming too much and he was losing sleep. Reluctantly, he pulled out and took another year away.

Dominic is well aware of his habitual patterns, his attitudes and his behaviours. But without support from others – either a network of colleagues or the system – this can only take you so far. And then another sort of guilt kicks in – of letting others down. 'I tend to burn out when I do things. I didn't want to blow it but ended up blowing it. Then I put myself down, call myself an idiot, interrogate myself about whether it is to do with being afraid of success, as one psychiatrist used to try telling me. But ultimately I don't buy that. Maybe it is to do with self-worth, but what I do know is I had very little support and I also know that this patient leadership lark can be very stressful at times. Let's not make it all about the individual – just as we should not make mental health problems all about the individual.'

Taking time out meant Dominic felt he had fallen behind somehow. This was exacerbated by coming off Twitter, his social support (itself a form of social media that can be volatile, polarised and 'triggering'). The King's Fund, which had commissioned the Barker work, 'Did not want to know any more. So I was a bit like "What's happening?" and I just did not hear back. I thought, "OK, I am not flavour of the month." That was tough to take.'

Again, we dwell on the swing between the necessary 'stepping up to challenge' and vulnerability to the reaction – particularly if the reaction is resonant of traumatic past experiences. 'I am either completely out there or will hide under the duvet.' Dominic pinpoints his drug experiences as providing the insight into these contradictory tendencies. 'If you use heroin, you have to be self-aware, as it is one of the most evil drugs out there. It is like another you in your head, trying to fool you into believing, for example, that you won't get hooked. You absolutely have to be hyper-vigilant.'

Dominic took a long holiday and looked after his mum, who had back problems. 'That is the least I can do. She has seen me go through hell and back.' He went back on social media, but realised that he would prefer to do more local work, where he could make more of a direct impact and where he saw change was desperately needed.

He helped develop a partnership forum that in turn drafted an involvement strategy for the local mental health trust. Through this he developed the more trusting relationships that all patient leaders need in order to influence the work. He helped secure senior commitment and resources to the ideas he espoused and felt good about it. Dominic was back. Again.

And Dominic's challenges were back. Again.

He was effectively project managing the emerging involvement strategy (as a volunteer) that led to the creation of a new role in the trust. He was led to believe that he might be able to job share this role and thus step back into work at his own pace and get off benefits. However, he lost out to someone who then became his manager and who didn't really know about co-production. But again, he did not give in, navigated a stormy period and came to chair a new partnership strategy group.

The group ensured that the trust funds 'people with lived experience' for their time and expertise – a hugely meaningful act in the patient leadership world. This was contentious, with some staff thinking patients should remain as volunteers. Dominic recalls one senior manager saying, 'I volunteer as a governor at a local school. Why don't they?' To which the response came from a service user: 'Yes, but you can afford to on £75,000 a year and you are healthy. You want inclusion? Pay me to come. I can barely afford to get to a GP appointment and am struggling with appealing my PIP [Personal Independence Payment], so there has to be something in it for me too.'

Dominic has felt the pushback from service users too – some complained that they would have sorted things out better but did not always come forward to try and help. 'I try to ignore that, rather than get irritated. But I also will make a stand if need be. I am learning that tricky balance, slowly!'

'Even now, I struggle to get to Cambridge. All the appointments I have are in the afternoon. I make reasonable adjustments and have got good people around me now.' (NB. A few days after this interview, Dominic became unwell again, though has since recovered.)

Dominic senses that this book, and how we are trying to model co-production in the writing of it, is one part of reclaiming the notion of patient leadership and its original intention – not to let it be co-opted, plagiarised and stolen from the people who have been part of the movement from the beginning, like Dominic himself. This is tricky, since the aim is to 'embed' it in the NHS.

But Dominic holds that too many people have taken the name without truly understanding what it is all about: 'Part of patient leadership is now about saying, "Hang on a minute, this is what patient leadership is, this is what it looks like."' He sees that this book is one element of that reclamation. 'It is a stake in the ground. This is who we are; this is our story of how it came about. You can't take that away from us, like some people and some organisations have tried to do.'

He tells a story of a well-known NHS commentator who puts out a regular blog that is read by thousands of staff. A few years back, this man came to speak at a regional conference on patient leadership. 'We, as service users, did not want him to come in the first place, but staff insisted – why should they always decide who comes? Turns out we were right.'

At the event, he was accused of misunderstanding entirely what patient leadership was about and seemed to alienate a lot of people in the audience: 'I was fuming, he said some appalling things, I thought he was a tosser. He did not have a clue.'

The book, to him, also feels like another attempt to pull people together. Dominic still needs the tribe. 'Just knowing there are people out there, even in the US and Canada, is a boost. People like me struggle with identity. Sometimes we don't know who we fucking are. We are lost. Discovering a new concept that helped position myself again has been amazingly important in my life, let alone the work. It's about identity, equality and power. It is who I am, who we are. It is a foundation for rebuilding our identity and integrity. I model myself on that. It takes a lot of self-confidence to even say that, but I do have a belief. I am worth that now.'

And like many, he has witnessed that his own experience in one part of the system is echoed in the experiences of others. He talks about Adam Bojelian, who lived until he was 15 with cerebral palsy, communicating only by blinking, and how his life was additionally scarred by prejudices concerning his disability and doctors making judgements about whether a life is worth living. 'He achieved so much; he was instrumental in bringing about NHS England policy changes: "When you are in the room don't shut the door, listen to me, I have an active brain with cerebral palsy." Now, that's real leadership. Let's smash those prejudices.' (For more information about Adam and the legacy of his

work, see http://intheblinkofaneyepoemsbyadambojelian.
blogspot.com.)

'It is amazing when I look back – we not only took the
notion of leadership on-board and tried to do stuff ourselves,
without any support from the system, but helped develop it,
clarify it, form it, take it to the next level. I've even written a
chapter in an academic book about it. I was the only person
without a PhD to be a contributor...though I did tell them I
had a degree in martial arts (which is true).' And there is that
twinkle again.

The issue of stigma is one he returns to. He is more open
about his mental health experiences than his drug past, as
he feels that disclosure can affect career opportunities. But
he is keen to put the story right and will always tend towards
speaking truth to power rather than shutting up. 'I've had
loads of different jobs when getting clean. I was a cashier,
putting money in the safe, and I was fine. But there are a
lot of preconceptions about what a drug addict is. I want to
break those down. When you think of a heroin addict, you
don't think of a big chap like I am nowadays!'

And again, we are back to the balance between doing the
work and looking after yourself – one that is of course a very
human one but is particularly acute for those who have been
affected by significant health problems: 'If I try to look after
myself too much I would not get anything done. Leadership
is about putting yourself out there.' And then, he poses the
question that seems to haunt all patient leaders: 'Can you
put yourself out there in a healthy way?' I have not heard
anyone articulate the problem so succinctly.

His advice to emerging patient leaders is simple but not

easy to take: 'Don't take on too much too quickly. That's the biggest mistake everyone makes. Don't try to be friends with everyone either, that's the trap, getting over-extended.' But we all do – that is the lure of the work.

Those of us who are sensitive about, and sensitised by, our experience have a vision of what good looks like and have 'skin in the game' to put it right. But integrity and vulnerability can come at a cost, particularly when it is not safe and when the role is unsupported compared with those available to professional leaders of change. I suggest to Dominic that perhaps that idealism and sensitivity is our blessing and our curse. He agrees.

And what of his messages for the system itself? He believes that lack of resources can be an excuse for poor care. 'It doesn't cost anything to be nice' – though he also admits staff are under lots of pressure. But he has seen that many in the system do not seem to be able to take negative feedback. He has seen this clearly more recently, as he has taken on the role of being an advocate for a family member. He knows that vulnerable people will always be scared of making concerns or complaints known. And for all these reasons, Dominic still puts himself in the firing line – or, to put it less militaristically, wants to be a bridge for improvement.

And he sees the difference when he is able to do this well – and when others around him, staff and patients/carers alike, work together. That is what keeps him going. His recent work on improving local emergency and urgent care services makes him smile with pride. On the back of the Barker Commission, his local area got funding to improve crisis care for people with mental health problems.

His project team, alongside the local mental health charity Mind, developed alternatives to going to A&E, a 'sanctuary' open 6pm–1am, a phone number where you could talk immediately to trained staff 24/7, nurses working alongside the police and last, but by no means least, in an NHS beset by IT systems that don't talk to each other, a shared information system between services.

'That is ground-breaking stuff, gritty work, and more important sometimes than that snazzy national stuff. I know it's a good service because I am using it and can see the changes.'

Having both been involved in various attempts to set up a national network for patient leaders, we believe that this sort of initiative needs to be patient led.

Given the dark forces that maintain the status quo, can patient leadership survive and thrive? 'Maybe it is just a fad,' I suggest. He disagrees vehemently. He jokes that his preferred title would be 'Jedi Master of Involvement'. I would be happy with that. After all, Jedis and *Star Wars* will be with us forever.

TRANSFORMERS

Sibylle Erdmann

We need to redefine what this work is. Every time I show up as a 'patient or carer' I dare to think that my presence is already a degree of disruption, creating some kind of change, opening up new possibilities.

The children, aged eight and six, open the door to me. One of them in a red ghoulish Halloween mask. Sibylle, their mum, offers me apple tart ('I would like to pretend that I made it myself, but a friend of mine did and brought it over earlier') and fresh coffee. The two boys settle down (eventually) to watch *Transformers*.

Sibylle comes over with two huge, A4, yellow ring binders that contain the children's voluminous records from their healthcare experiences: 'We got really good at filing and record-keeping. One of the skills you have to develop and continually practise when caring for those you love with long-term ill health.' There are other reasons for how the parents have pulled through after almost a decade of looking after their two children with complex healthcare needs. But for Sibylle, it seems to begin and end with support – not something that everyone has during tough times when worlds fall apart.

More than that, Sibylle is now a champion for the voice of parents and children in hospitals – for those born with the sort of devastating early complications of both her children due to premature birth. She has become someone who supports other parents and staff on how to work together as a team, campaigning for greater involvement of parents in medical decision-making, for instance by attending ward rounds. Drawing attention to this next generation of patients, Sibylle has gone on to be a national champion for an emerging network of national 'patient leaders'.

In her everyday life as a parent carer, with her children now at school age, she strives beyond healthcare to the integration of children with healthcare needs into mainstream schools, a fight she maintains has been every bit as hard as the one she has had to fight for her kids in hospital. In this work, Sibylle makes use of the professional skills she has acquired as a teacher and organisational consultant, even though the official role she is often introduced as having is 'mum'.

'When our first son was born at 24 weeks, far too early, we had to spend over a year in hospital with him. There were many complications and setbacks. We lived from one day to the next for 400 days on various wards. With time slowed down, we had to live in the moment. Even though life was dampened, it paradoxically turned into a time of clarity, a space beyond words, almost hauntingly beautiful.'

This reflective space and a sense of living very much in the now is something that Sibylle comes back to time and time again in our conversations: 'I found myself questioning what I was thinking and doing. I went back to things I had not done since I was a child – making things and also making *sense* of things.' Before having children, Sibylle had an intense job that involved working many office hours, constant travelling for business and being there for clients. She says: 'I really enjoyed my work. That was the role I concentrated on – my primary role, a professional role.'

It is hard to reconcile the changes and the struggles of this family with the easy-going nature of the household I am witnessing this afternoon. The two boys are very excited at the thought of the book (they want to be chapter four by the way). Sibylle at one stage during our conversation is asked to make a helmet for a toy out of orange cardboard. She obliges. Their life seems a continuous bustle of boyish energy. The two kids go back to making dens and watching TV.

Sibylle goes back to her story and her time in hospital. As with many in crisis, perspectives about priorities came to the fore: 'What's in and what's out. It is a time when you come to realise what is important and what is not. Just being a parent is hard enough – being hospitalised changed things even more radically.'

Parents with a child born too early find themselves living in this neonatal world, and they have to find new ways of bonding with the child. Of creating a private enclave in this public hospital environment. Sibylle feels that they managed as well as they could with 15-hour visits to hospital every day, a family island created out of a physio mat on the floor and as many children's books as they could possibly delve into. In the absence of any physical changes, they surrounded themselves with stories. 'We managed to create a live world with a one-metre radius.'

Her relationships with others in the neonatal wards became close and often supportive. She shows me photos from the hospital days – of the matron smiling beatifically out of the old print, a nurse who made a special 15 minutes of time at the end of every ten-hour shift to come and hug the baby.

These experiences hold clues for the sort of 'transformer' she was herself to become – someone always looking for spaces that allow a different type of knowing, different modes of expression and the relational over the transactional, 'So I can make a real contribution in that parent space.'

Her experiences on the neonatal unit, surrounded by life-and-death decisions and by intimate love and support within a heroic yet alienating technological environment, explain her search for different ways of seeing – a hallmark of a patient leader. Sibylle is deeply interested in the 'kind of voice' that gives meaning about human relations and connections. Where do you turn when nothing makes sense, the world has tipped upside down and dreams and futures have been battered?

Within this need to remake meaning comes the way for disentanglement from the wreckage. This is a territory that is often unwritten about – where a patient or carer finds the tools they need from deep within themselves. And it is hardly surprising that at this point one leans into professional or life expertise.

Both Sibylle and her husband had worked in organisational consulting – they knew how organisations work and had learned how to ask questions for the benefit of an agreed outcome: 'In the hospital environment, it is easy to feel passive and infantilised, but it was our survival mechanism not to succumb to that. We tried to understand the questions we needed to ask. We were building up our credibility by participating, being helpful. So as to be equals in the care for our child, knowing that we would be taking on this care for the rest of our lives. This was about regaining power and allowing our way of knowing into the system.'

And in the regaining of power, there was also a need to reframe the conversation, to retrieve the human from the purely medical.

Sibylle is benevolent but crystal clear in her challenge to the well-meaning but at times limiting approaches that she has encountered in this healthcare journey. And the contribution that families can make on the ward and also at a strategic level.

In the more progressive neonatal hospital wards, parents are taught how to be involved as carers – equipped to take care of the tubes, drugs and paraphernalia that will accompany them for a while, sometimes for a lifetime. However, as Sibylle points out gently: 'This is only one part of our role. We parents don't just want to be trained as carers, we also want to be mum and dad. We need to be able to have a medical engagement as well as a parental connection with our child. When looking at our child, we want to know how to check for clues of being unwell. Yet, we also want to just see our baby, a new addition in an extended family.'

And sometimes, as Sibylle recalls, there are just plain battles with healthcare professionals, when you have to take sides. She has anecdotes of stepping in to prevent an intervention from happening or making one happen. As parents, it is possible to be treated as equal partners on the ward. But one wonders how many do not get to this point, or do not have the professional expertise, articulacy or support.

In her work today as an educator and improver, Sibylle often draws on the experiences she lived through in that time. She comes with concrete and pragmatic examples of the kind of healthcare issues she encountered. She is a strong believer that life experiences and real stories can highlight the urgency of a need for change.

One of the issues that comes up time and time again for different patients and carers is the fragmentation across the healthcare system. Sibylle always found it quite illuminating to recount to healthcare teams what a typical series of outpatient appointments can look like in practice. 'Every body part is seen by a different hospital or department that often don't interlink with each other at best or even have in-fighting.' The human body is dissected into various parts. Parents are playing the central role of coordination, which is demanding. Healthcare workers in one part of the system often don't get to hear what it's like at the other part and how it hangs together (or not) from the patient perspective.

With this bank of experiences, Sibylle has built up a vast knowledge store that can be brought to bear. I ask her, half in jest, about who the best medical professionals are. She takes me by surprise again – is unequivocal: 'Anaesthetists have a way of knowing. They are the frontliners who read the situation, tell the truth and say the right thing – what needs to be said.' 'This seems all about trust,' I say. 'Yes. I came to trust different people differently.'

'And where are surgeons on the list?' I ask mischievously, assuming they might sometimes tend to want to do an operation. Sibylle knows a thing or two about tact though and avoids an answer.

There are other silos that are hard to break down as kids age – from neonatal to paediatrics, to children and young people's services, to those for adults. This sort of advocacy is for the long haul.

'You are well supported while you are still in hospital. But about a third of those who go through neonatal departments have long-term differences, for example with their vision, hearing, cerebral palsy, whatever.' Families can become weary, lonely, unpaid care coordinators: 'It's hard to bring people, staff and teams together. It's all about negotiating and keeping going, and ultimately the question is, how do we "hand over" to the kids to speak for themselves eventually?'

We pause before Sibylle refers to their second child, a chatty six-year-old who is still learning to walk and covering longer distances in a wheelchair. The community-based support is haphazard and unstable, with therapists rotating fast in their roles.

We talk about visible and invisible disabilities and the implications for taking part in public life. And the ignorance and stigma associated with both. 'It takes much lobbying to address the fears of any institution around different abilities, how to welcome differences and learn from them.'

Sibylle recounts many frustrating experiences along the way of closed doors, mindless policies, no-go areas for no reason and unnecessary binary thinking. With disability, you are often finding yourself in the position to ask for 'permission to participate', always having to check the small print. Always wondering whether there will be a lift, always wondering whether it will be working.

Healing is not a linear path, and for those patient leaders who take up the task of trying to help improve and transform healthcare, it is a twisting route that veers between the personal and the professional and can double back on itself in terms of remission and relapse.

For Sibylle, who has been campaigning for the health and societal integration of her own and other children for a decade, healing is all about growth and learning. She is writing her doctorate thesis on this. She is keen to make something of the experience. Sibylle's studies on organisational change augment her personal wisdom: 'The more I study organisations and how change can occur, the more I realise it's not only about marching for a cause but also about coming together differently.' As a way to process her experiences and, frankly, worries of not knowing, she would often wake at 5am to write, reflect and busy her thoughts.

'It was hard at first to demarcate my own time, create a boundary with just me in it, as I spent most of the time thinking about my family.' Her studies took her on a trip abroad while her sick two-year-old was cared for by the dad, and she, ultimately, thought that it would be a healthy sign that her child could be safe and well without her. All was fine and, in fact, the child started to walk in this time of 'mummy being away'. As she puts it, 'This was my price to pay not to witness that. After being hospital bound for so long, it took me some time to justify any distances – how far can I go?'

When taking her private stories into the public space, giving talks at hospitals or conferences, she was surprised at how 'patient and carer stories' provide an implicit permission to display emotions and to be vulnerable for everyone in the room. These stories give permission to bring the personal into the space.

Sibylle is taking the skill of public speaking that she honed in her professional life and translating it into a new way of presenting herself. And many other patient advocates who are in a similar situation do exactly the same thing: teachers, artists, designers, project managers and accountants use their skills and their knowledge as public agents and bring it together with their private sphere. Because this kind of private experience is complemented by an understanding of what the public demands are. 'With our children, we are constantly asked to re-present ourselves: in front of the doctor, at the school, in the lift. These are all public appearances of an otherwise private unit. The public and the private are deeply enmeshed.'

Parent advocacy in the neonatal world is becoming well established and is ahead of other fields. In the neonatal setting, the patient and the patient advocate are two different people. This is a unique situation, which enables learning about patient advocacy and applying it more widely. More-over, most neonatal units now work in networks, with strong governance structures that include the voice of the parent. There is formal recognition that the insights and feedback from parents is valuable from a strategic and operational perspective.

But advocacy and patient leadership are not 'a cause' for Sibylle. She offers a more pragmatic sense of the work to be undertaken. And this *is* work even though for some health-care staff patient engagement rarely constitutes work. It is the link between the personal and the professional that is crucial: 'We need to redefine what this work is. Every time I show up as a "patient or carer" I dare to think that my presence is already a degree of disruption, creating some kind of change, opening up new possibilities. I am invited to be at the table, I am invited to comment.' With this, of course, comes the question of how valuing this kind of work is expressed – what kind of remuneration would be fair? – a complex and contentious topic for many patient leaders.

A big part of Sibylle's work is sharing stories. 'I have been recounting my private experiences, making use of anec-dotes in the hope that they are memorable to others, giving a personal interpretation of the impact of healthcare work. What I now find is that I am equally collating anecdotes about how my patient stories resonate. For every story told, I get a story in return. For instance, I gave a speech to a large audience of quality improvers about being a parent carer. At the end of my speech one of the organisers commented on how "good it was to hear from someone who was not a professional". It struck me that this was the first time in my adult life that I was called "not a professional". It made me wonder what I now was. If not a professional – what was the opposite of that? What is this kind of work if it is not seen as professional?' Sibylle says she did some casual research into what people thought was the opposite of 'professional' and got back all sorts of responses.

Recently, when Sibylle spoke in front of thousands of doctors at a major international conference, she was asked to be part of a panel discussion with three medical specialists. A friend in the audience later told her that she did well and 'held her ground' while on stage. Which is – if you had to sum it up – the core of the work of a patient advocate. We are holding our ground, demarcating the boundaries. Because we are not operating out of roles but speaking from our identities. 'It was surprising to hear that this "work" of ground holding was visible to the entire audience. It is actually exactly what I am doing, whether on stage or in the medical appointment.' I am aware that, though fitting, the metaphor is defensive and binary. It is winning by not losing. I long for the day that this battle is not apparent any longer.

Sibylle tells me how she shows pictures of her sons' art (see below) as a backdrop during conferences and they are delighted to be known as artists, rather than through a passive 'patient' lens. Sibylle is one of several patient/carer leaders who care deeply about the concepts behind what they do. For her it's as much about how you present yourself or 're-present' yourself that matters. Perhaps this is the meaning that should underpin the notion of 're-presentation'.

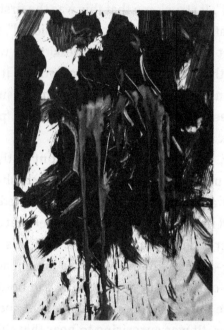

Beginnings – first representation of the world

To the question of how she makes a difference, Sibylle gives an elaborate answer: 'In this patient leadership world I am looking for changes in paradigm rather than outcomes measured in metrics. I am not looking for a straightforward causality. I can only know what I am doing differently in my own sphere. I can build alliances with other people and see what works, hoping for a small change.'

'I have personal metrics of success, such as being invited to attend a meeting where no service user has been before, having a platform to speak in front of a healthcare audience (often with the generous brief to say whatever I see fit), to eventually feel welcome in a meeting where at first nobody wanted to sit next to me for fear I might be too "other". I see success when healthcare experts reach out to me, seeking my advice and input into their models, programmes, publications. There is also success in making connections through the conversations with other parents, where we usually come out nodding at the recognition of the themes that are brought to the table, encouraged to keep on talking about these themes in our respective public and social realms.'

Sibylle acknowledges that, as a parent and not as a 'patient', she is more in a position of observer, always working with 'transmitted pain' as she dubs it (that of a carer rather than the person who receives care). Whether or not this is easier is uncertain. As a mental health service user, my decisions were always made through a filter of guilt and shame about how others felt. And perhaps the difference between 'patient' and 'carer' leaders can be explored another time.

Whatever the truth (maybe there isn't one), we come back to the assertion that patient and carer leaders tap into different ways of knowing. This is what Sibylle is all about – that and her instinctive generosity and curiosity. For her, 'knowing flows into doing', and this is where, she admits, 'I can be at my best.'

'If I ever get angry when I hear healthcare professionals say, "Patients have no knowledge," that infers all knowledge is in medicine, that patients are inferior, but we as people, and as different professionals or with our own experiences, bring other forms of knowledge.'

If all this makes Sibylle sound overly theoretical, she is far from it: 'Humour is important. I got through all the episodes of *Friends*, in times of serious distress – I just couldn't stand the news or serious documentaries. I watched stupid films. I still do. I'm not embarrassed! This is also part of supporting yourself in difficult times. Nourish yourself, trust what you know, have conversations and connect with others.'

By the time we have finished talking, it's dark outside. As I leave, I ask her how she finds the energy to carry on after a decade. 'It's in the everyday. It's about showing up, making the change in the moment, saying, "This is odd, why do it this way...?"'

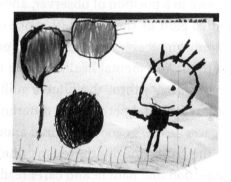

Child in the park, playing ball under the sunshine

CRUMBS FROM THE TABLE

Alison Cameron

I was the only 'patient'... There were hundreds of staff, and me. We had to put Post-its on a wall, yuk. But I suddenly thought: 'I have the right to be included...' This is what I wrote on my Post-it: 'I have the RIGHT to be here.'

If there is one characteristic to describe all the patient leaders in this book – my gang of friends, and many others who I have met – it is 'authenticity'. The capacity, or perhaps the internal demand of the will, to be 'authentic'. Perhaps it becomes almost a duty for patient leaders to bring that authenticity into influencing change – having been through so much, having survived and then made the choice to struggle for what is right, you have to bring 'all of yourself' into the work.

And Alison Cameron, for me, is the epitome of 'authenticity'. It seems to be her huge gift but also a terrible burden at times.

Thus, the crushing insight that she had 'ceased to care' was the moment she realised 'how spiritually ill' she had become.

Alison is one of the brightest and most intelligent people I have ever met. How did she come to struggle so much in her life? What brought her to the point of being a 'healthcare icon' for many of us in the mental health and patient leadership movement, yet still so marginalised by a system that does not seem able to find a way of working with people like her?

She patiently explains the threads. Her job in international relations coordinating humanitarian activities meant everything to her. 'That career became my identity; I didn't do anything else. I was fresh out of university but was already challenging much of what I saw and the assumptions people made. It was always about making a difference while working in partnership with communities.'

She contrasts this to what she saw around her. For others it seemed more about wielding power. This translated to a 'patronising, and rather colonial, willingness to help, but only on their terms – "We know what is best for these people" – and an expectation that those on the receiving end should be grateful for our largesse.'

'Wherever I went – whether in the Chernobyl zone of Belarus after the nuclear accident or Zimbabwe – I didn't see victims but people with huge strengths who could help themselves. What we needed to do was invest in capacity building, allowing them to decide their own solutions.'

The problem was that this idealism, sensitivity and insight – plus the raw need to speak truth to power – was at odds with the culture within which she worked. So, she was alone. Something that is all too familiar nowadays in her work as a patient leader.

This sort of insight is tough to bear. It was made more difficult because Alison was also struggling with anxiety and depression and had been for many years before her work in international development. She did manage to create opportunities for people, and she kept going because of her 'devotion' to the individuals she met despite being trapped in what she perceived as an extremely bullying culture that emanated from the chief executive and cascaded throughout the entire organisation.

'I was a breakdown waiting to happen. I was ill for a long time and kept going and pushing beyond my limits, because of my devotion to the communities with which I was working.'

And then two of her colleagues were killed in a horrific accident in Belarus – caught in the propellers of a boat that had just turned on its engine. They had been in the water together after a drunken gathering.

Alison was despatched to sort things out and visit the mortuary (without refrigeration in 34-degree heat) and then felt immense pressure over how to handle the court proceedings because of the potential scandal – several politicians had been at the party: 'My boss had been dismembered. My other colleague drowned. They found 15 other corpses – not connected to this incident – when they dredged the river.'

The full breakdown came in 1998. 'I was asked a simple question during a work meeting that I knew the answer to. But something in me froze. I had ceased to care. The bullying environment and effects of the death of a colleague seemed to have cut me off from my principles and values. I had the sensation of not giving a damn. Of withdrawing into an inner passivity. I went back to my office, packed up my desk and went home. I didn't go back.'

The conflict between her need for authenticity in her role and the surrounding work culture were too much. On top of this now came a crushing sense of inner withdrawal from both her 'caring' self and loss of work identity: 'I could not envisage not having that identity any more. The impact of having to accept that this identity was gone was devastating.'

After a year on sick pay, she recovered enough to get a job running the Moscow School of Economics' office in Moscow State University. She did not realise how ill she was, and, alone in a strange city, she quickly became too ill to work. Even during that time, she managed to get another job working for a Member of the European Parliament (MEP). She found herself temporarily in accommodation in Chelsea: 'I tried to take my own life for the first time in my landlady's house. She was a leading light of the Chelsea pro-life movement. I nicked her gin. She had to throw me out.'

She was now homeless and entered what she describes as her 'twilight zone' where she was under the radar for any meaningful support.

She self-medicated with alcohol: 'I was drinking myself to death, because I had "died" with my identity gone and couldn't go back. What else did I have? I obliterated my brain, went in and out of hospital and psychiatric wards. I was gone, beyond feeling anything at all, and I stayed in that state for a long time.'

'I was in and out of hospital, getting scraped off the pavement. They thought I had rapid recycling bipolar as I was in every two weeks. My benefits came every two weeks, so I would run out of money, experience withdrawal. I was in hostels, homeless crisis units, you name it, I've been there.'

As with many patient leaders, she witnessed at first hand the incredible disconnection between services. She fell through many cracks. Polite conversations in policy-making circles about the need for 'integration' pale when considering the sometimes-devastating consequences of continuity gone wrong.

'A file went missing between a social worker, the mental health team and the homeless unit. It was about how vulnerable I was. I didn't get to the homeless unit, so none of what was crucial was considered. I ended up with all my possessions in a black bin liner. I was packed off to an illegally converted building in Tottenham, miles away from any support. I couldn't go on the tube, I was disoriented.'

Alison was hauled into a neighbour's flat and raped. She only just escaped, 'by remembering how to say something in Arabic that I had learned from a foreign office briefing!'

Using 'stories' is now part of the NHS lexicon. But some stories are more profound than others: 'When I talk to NHS folk, I ask them to think about it: this was one file; one tiny part of a process map that people draw on a flip chart in posh seminars about quality improvement. This was simply a breakdown between teams. But the teams never see the person between the teams, in that gap. They do not see the consequences of what they do. Be aware: the decision you make has human consequences.'

But she is also wise to the emotional consequences of sharing, disclosing, being vulnerable and being 'authentic': 'Telling this takes a lot out of me. It retraumatises me. But the double bind is that if it doesn't take a lot out of me, then I am not talking about it with integrity, I am just in my head. I have to feel the authenticity.' She tries now to use her stories 'judiciously' with those who are 'ready to hear it'.

The struggle to get back into life was enormous. 'My assumption was that my useful life was over. I stumbled into a service user meeting of my local branch of Mind. I met a rather grand lady in pearls in the ladies.'

They got talking about dual diagnosis and the problems of two different systems being unable to work collaboratively. The 'posh lady' turned out to be the chair of Central and North West London NHS Foundation Trust. Alison was called in to join various local NHS committees.

I ask her: 'Apart from not mislaying files, what could anyone have done to make things easier?' She answers: 'It would be nice if services spoke to one another. I spent such a long time in the "revolving door". A plea for coordination seems so simplistic. Also: ask me what I think! Then I might not have had such a hard time.'

During a month-long period that she does not remember, she was stabbed and subsequently discovered by a local pastor who'd left a note in her bag: 'I don't remember it. I had gone blank because my already traumatised brain could not take in any more. I was found in Archway in a psychotic state, dressed smartly, happy as Larry, immortal, imagining angels would take me to another planet.' There was good reason for this delusional episode. She could not remember anything about being stabbed. Her feverish temperature had triggered the delirium.

Alison had assumed her professional and political lives were over, but she very slowly realised that there was a way of turning something terrible into something positive. 'That was really important to me.'

At a meeting, she heard Rachel Perkins, a clinical psychologist who had been diagnosed as bipolar, a powerful advocate of people with mental health problems and a pioneer in the service user movement. Rachel had found ways in her organisation, what is now South West London and St George's Mental Health NHS Trust, to employ people with mental health problems. This was the 'seed' – the idea that a different path towards a professional and influential life was possible. 'It was important to hear that I might be able to work again, and this started me on the path of getting involved.'

The next surprise was that a few people were starting to listen to what Alison had to say about her experiences. Then the surreal nature of her professional life began to unfold. On one level, she struggled to exist. Jobless, still ill, vulnerable. But 'wheeled in', as she puts it, to say things that others could not.

'I went with two of my own psychiatric nurses from my ward to speak at a King's Fund training event on acute care. So, here I was telling them the reality of how I was considered too mad for substance misuse services and too drunk for mental health services. I talked about disconnection while I floated between their world and mine. While they were eating duck à l'orange. As the biscuits floated by.'

And at a deep level, the relationship she was building was with herself: 'I could reconnect with what I used to do – talking to and being listened to, having a voice and planting seeds. I can see when people get the point I am trying to make. I can see the penny drop, the light bulb light up. These moments are priceless.'

One day, when helping to launch a report, she stepped slightly out of line, once more speaking truth to power. She was a speaker at the launch of a report on training staff. 'I said there's no point in training frontline staff if psychiatrists further up the ladder aren't interested. There was an audible murmur: "Oh I don't like this criticism of psychiatrists." But then someone important from the Royal College of Psychiatrists, in this posh voice, came out with: "I have to agree with what that woman said. Most of my colleagues are more interested in clinical excellence awards than anything else."'

The courageous Alison was (partly) back: 'I was saying what was obvious but realised then that I had the power to say stuff that other people think but never dare to actually say.' She was asked back and was invited to several local and national events; her humour, sharpness of articulation and self-deprecation were infectious (in this author's view).

Alison often refers to a book by the pioneering Edgar Cahn called *No More Throw-Away People: The Co-Production Imperative*. She understood the message in the book that everyone considered 'useless' for whatever reason – illness, old age, disability, etc. – has something to contribute.

From her work with a London-based day centre for which Edgar Cahn was an advisor, she started using the term 'frozen assets'. She often uses that image when discussing co-production and user involvement: 'At this time, these assets I had had – an urgent need to be authentic, a compelling desire to support people, a need to speak honestly – these things were starting to thaw out a bit.'

But the patient leader can be a perennial outsider. 'To begin with, it was great. I got lunch here and there. I did feel grateful. But at the same time, I had no permission to be part of something. I dreamt once of a Chagall-like stained glass window. I was on the outside, looking through it at everyone on the inside. I could not get in, so I stayed pressed against the glass.'

Gradually, confidence and a bit of stability returned. She had turned to Alcoholics Anonymous (AA) and was gaining a sense of self-worth. The journey should have been smooth from then on. It hasn't been. 'I started to think, "Hang on. I am being parachuted in to face those with the power." I was waiting for power. I am still waiting.'

With that returning sense of self-validity came the regained insight: 'I was expected to be grateful for crumbs from the table.'

Frustrated with inequalities of access to having a voice in healthcare leadership – in turn mirroring what she was experiencing at service level – she found herself once again in the invidious and isolated position of speaking truth to power in a closed environment.

'I never felt like I belonged in those professional groups. I was being told how inspirational I was, but nothing changed.

I inspired people, made them cry, got a biscuit and a cup of tea, was patted on the head and sent on my way. If anything did happen, I was never a part of it.'

The deep resonance of exclusion and unfairness is never far from the surface of patient leaders. It resonates twice, in fact – at the level of what has happened as a user of services (and, I would add as a personal opinion, I think this happens particularly frequently for those with mental health problems), and it may resonate at a deeper, personal level for those who have experienced other trauma. And without any system for supporting patient leaders and without peer support, relapse and illness are not far off.

'I had PTSD [post-traumatic stress disorder]. I didn't know how to manage the emotional connection. It would only take some small interaction on some committee to replicate some of the things that happened before, and I would go into emotional overwhelm. I could be very angry.'

She knows that it must be hard for staff to be on the receiving end of what may seem like disproportionate anger. 'I had had no therapy. I could put on a polished facade of being well at times, even when profoundly unwell.' And with stunning insight, she adds: 'That's always been another aspect of me – trying not to lose control. I would and do overdo it. So, I come across as wanting to take over the world, when actually I felt like a pile of crap.'

There were a few people she was drawn to during these periods of climbing, people she reckons 'planted more seeds' – such as a young doctor in A&E who'd been up all night who looked after her and teasingly called her a 'maelstrom of mayhem', but in Alison's mind recognised her immense struggle to re-find her strength.

AA was a sanctuary, as well. As Alison's a natural storyteller, it's best to hear her description of what happened there: 'First meeting, I was under the influence slightly. I didn't know what to expect. It's a posh area (I am always homeless in posh areas. I had standards to maintain). I listened to a film director, feeling offended that he swore. They slowed down the meeting for newcomers. They must mean me. I need to get approval. I spoke: "I am Alison and I am an alcoholic." I had not seen myself as that and something lifted a bit, a bit. I am such a drama queen, so I would like to have had stigmata and angels trumpeting at that moment, but it was just a light lifting and something that had been absent coming in.' She waves the moment away, ever doubtful: 'This was cheesy, but it was hope, definitely. It probably started then. Like when the Wizard of Oz moves from black and white to colour.'

She found other allies during a patient leadership training course in 2010. This is where we first met. At this time, she was becoming more involved in health service improvement work in north-west London, and, though it was a struggle, she felt she could start to tackle the anger and contradictory passions she felt in her work to improve healthcare. 'I must have been ready – when the pupil is ready, the teacher will appear. I was lucky even to have survived.'

Other moments came, though they seemed fleeting. Alison had not found her tribe yet. But amongst health professionals who welcomed her in, she sensed possibility. 'Once, I did a horrible group exercise when I was the only "patient" doing a postgraduate course at the NHS Leadership Academy. There were hundreds of staff, and me. We had to put Post-its on a wall, yuk. But I suddenly thought: "I have the right to be included, inside the church." This is what I wrote on my Post-it: "I have the RIGHT to be here.""

Being included. Being excluded. This swing is common for many. Alison's experiences with national organisations in the ensuing years meant this swing felt particularly wild. She had a contract with NHS England, during which time she often felt included – being part of large, patient-led initiatives and teams – for which she remains grateful. But at other times she felt excluded.

'That was hard. It is sometimes an advantage not to be within. People often use me to challenge others because they are too scared in their role to do so. This could help in shifting power. The assumption that we have no power if we are at the edge of things is not always true, but it doesn't make for a settled life, that's for sure.'

She adds: 'I move from feeling powerful to powerless many, many times during the day, weeks, months and years. Sometimes I don't want to be part of the establishment because I then have to give up on myself. But I yearn to be part of a team, to be a worker among workers, a friend among friends. I don't want to be a special case or a token patient to show how co-productive we are.'

In my own opinion, without a true, big gang – a network, call it what you will, but something that provides a wider sense of loose belonging – patient leaders will always suffer from this ambivalence to being included as part of the system's efforts to improve things.

Caught within my own train of thought, I ask: 'Do we need our own gang?' This is not an easy question for any of us. She addresses the question tentatively: 'It would help, but it is not a panacea. It would be useful for those at an earlier stage, definitely – a source of support, particularly for those in that angry place when you're invited to NHS meetings to tick the box.'

Of all patient leaders, I feel that Alison is the one who has thought most about this need for a gang. But she is also aware that our heterogeneity is a strength. She does not want to create a separate box. The main thing is about helping each other: 'The key is to have a shared space for learning and working – being able to identify ways to work with people and systems that are not ready for the change we envisage. A place where we can regather our strength.'

Steeped in Eastern European history, Alison has dubbed patient leaders as 'quiet revolutionaries' and sees historical parallels in what this social movement needs. While the notion of 'revolution' implies a sense of taking control 'over' others, she is clear that this is not what we are doing – it is more about equalising power. But to get there, of course, things need to change.

Her experience of working with NHS England and other national agencies, she says, reveals an inability for health-care systems to move beyond minimal forms of engagement, such as consultation, feedback and having a few represent-atives on committees: 'It is great up to a point, but even current adaptations of the ladder of engagement [Arnstein 1969] leave out the need for improvement and change to be truly patient or citizen led. What is stopping that from hap-pening? That's the question. I think that's the barrier. That sort of thinking requires a real power shift.'

Meanwhile, it is where patient leaders do work directly

with staff that she remains staunchly convinced that it is not a fight for takeover and control. Her experience is not used to knock professionals over the head. Instead, she sees staff who are under pressure too: 'I am not justifying lapses in care, but I can see mistakes made when people are under such severe pressure in work situations.'

She doesn't buy into the sort of 'resilience' training handed down by NHS HR departments and, like many patient leaders, is eager to work with professionals and systems to find other solutions: 'I know it's easy to get cut off from compassion. It can happen to anybody and I see it regularly in healthcare.' 'In other words,' she says, 'patient leaders just see things from a different angle and could help.'

I push Alison on whether she has seen any hints of a shift in thinking in her years of being involved with staff who are trying to improve services. She is keen to point to local initiatives where people have worked in more collaborative ways, adapting different ways to value people (e.g. Timebanks) and where users and citizens have had more say in solutions, rather than just being 'feedback fodder'.

But the changes she sees are still at the margins. Maybe it is just early days, I suggest. Whatever the answer, Alison is determined to keep her own authenticity, but it still comes at a cost that few recognise: 'This work damages my health. It is often not done in a supportive working environment. It is about more than giving me a job description. It is me bringing bits of myself, offering that generously, hoping that contributes. But I am not sure others can cope with that. But if I am merely someone who is "involved" and learns the lingo and adjusts to the system (like most patients do at the individual level), then what difference is there? What change is that modelling? That we have to adapt (again)?'

Overall, Alison, like many others, is offering a way to 'expand the field of vision', as she puts it. 'My job – my "mission" if you like – I think is to bring authenticity and a permission to allow people to use their ability to think in a totally different way, away from the intellect where all that process stuff sits and allow for others a way into emotion and vulnerability. Because I know how dangerous it is to be cut off from that due to the toxic nature of the work environment.'

This message is not just for staff. She has witnessed people she once considered 'patient leaders' morph into 'system people'. She states: 'I despair as I hear systems speak. There is a loss there, of authentic experience, being brutally honest about these things and laying bare a vulnerability – something powerful in that it enables people to reconnect with their "difficult stories".'

She talks about how she has been part of intense work within a senior managers' leadership programme. Here, her role was to present her story in a challenging and dramatic way in order to delve deeply into how people responded. Also, to work with what Alison was going through while 'opening up'. They explored how it was very easy for people in the room to distract themselves by talking in terms of generalities and policy formulation rather than working with the difficult feelings this brought up.

Alison tells the story of how one senior manager burst into tears, not because of the power of Alison's story, but because she saw clearly how she had had to cut herself off from her own feelings to manage in the job she had. 'She had negated this person she had been. This was a painful realisation and had a knock-on effect in the room – something unlocked in her and us. She then felt the courage to come right out with how she felt.'

So, it is about 'patients' bringing people back to their humanness? 'Yes, yes, something about that is intensely powerful. But I also have to manage my energy. It has to be delivered in a supportive environment. I then get filled up as well as drained. What drains me is an unsafe working environment. Because then I am exposing myself to such an extent.'

Alison sees good intent in many NHS individuals, but that 'many who work in "patient and public engagement" have not thought things through properly'. In other words, what Alison is saying is that the system and individuals within it still habitually cut off from the difficult work of true patient leadership. It not only threatens the system and status quo, but also their own built-up habitual defences against being more human. She agrees with this way of seeing it.

Much of the work she has done with the NHS Leadership Academy has been constructive, and she has found herself crying 'for good reasons' during and after the sessions she helps to deliver there. 'I have joy for these future leaders who have understood something deeply from what I have said. They haven't been got at yet; the system hasn't drained them yet. They will come up and tell me stuff – expose the reason why they joined the NHS, talk of their mental health problems, even addiction.' She is waiting for wider leadership in healthcare circles to come to terms with the balance between personal vulnerability and leadership and thinks patient leaders can help if there are more opportunities for them at senior level.

Ultimately, Alison feels she can 'almost handle it' if she sees change as a result. But too often, she still sees habitual defensiveness at system and personal levels. And she sees too many leaders in the NHS keeping their heads below the parapet, either about the need for change or about toxic cultures.

Alison continues her struggle with both mental and physical health problems and has found it difficult to find work and to risk coming off benefits.

But she is reconnecting with her former life and interests (she is a talented writer and has begun blogging about her experiences). She has renewed her old relationships with friends from Belarus, enjoys speaking Russian and reading poetry (she was close friends with Vera Rich, a well-known poet, literary translator and human rights campaigner) and continues to support friends and strangers – including people without support in psychiatric hospitals.

And as she reconnects, she continues to have a huge influence on other patient leaders and NHS staff – as a presenter, strategist, advocate and social media influencer. And more importantly, to me anyway, as a friend who has been there from the very Winchester beginnings and still believes in the power of patient leadership.

There seems no chance of Alison being able to give up her authenticity these days, though those of us who love her continue to worry about her during her dark times. I have seen the huge strides Alison has made, but she often cannot see those. However, she now acknowledges that she deserves more, that some individuals and organisations are 'not worth killing myself over'.

She warns others not to be naive: 'When I emerged on

the scene, I was treated as a commodity. Everyone wanted a bit of me.' She describes a scene after a big NHS event when two representatives from national agencies descended on her, claiming responsibility for 'discovering' her. 'I was pulled towards one stand and I could hear this other woman calling, "She was with my team first."'

Often, bitter experience has taught her not to be quite so ready to believe the lofty promises of NHS leaders requiring a chunk of her to boost their own egos. 'Being a patient leader requires the growing of a thick skin. I found working with national NHS bodies and the think-tank world corrosive at times and I had long ago lost my protective armour.'

Beneath the immense strength that Alison reveals, like all patient leaders she is still vulnerable: 'It was very easy to hurt me, as I cared so much but my skin was paper thin. My health suffered badly as a result. We need support, and we need clarity as to what is expected of us, particularly if ill health has kept us out of the workforce for an extended period. It is not enough just to parachute us in. The NHS world is unique and can be rather unhealthy, a fact to which I can personally attest. I look forward to regaining my health, my strength and my ability to speak truth to power, even if my voice shakes.'

Reference

Arnstein, S. R. (1969) 'A ladder of citizen participation.' *Journal of the American Planning Association* 35, 4, 216–224.

WALKING THE TALK

David Festenstein

I've got underneath the car with this... One clinician...said: 'I will never see a patient in the same way again.' I was very excited; I began to call it my 'stroke of luck'; it was opening up such fascinating opportunities. I was so pumped, and, as I talk about it, despite the frustrations that came later, there is still so much to share.

'I celebrated being able to peel open a banana,' David laughs.

This, from someone who had been a successful communications expert, his world turned upside down by a massive stroke in his 50s.

Maybe it was his communications background that helped him through. Certainly, throughout our conversations, it is a clear articulation about what he learned from his experience, an attention to what was going on internally and externally and his vision of being able to help others, that led to his extraordinary adjustment to his own earthquake.

And it is perhaps this clear vision that allows him also to see how good his care has been and how poor the NHS is at learning from patients – in particular being able to draw on patient-led innovation.

But back to those small things: 'I felt grateful for being able to put the toothpaste top back on the tube. Being able to walk from here to there.' He is pointing to the window two metres away.

In the summer of 2008, David had been burying his beloved cat ('It used to sit under my desk for hours') and attributed his 'not feeling quite right' to jet lag after a holiday in Chicago. After developing pins and needles, he suddenly felt much more unwell and scared. After recovering slightly, he phoned his wife and told her he had done something to his back.

She drove him to hospital, saying later that she had noticed his drooping right arm all the way in the car. But on finding he could not undo his seat belt, he merely reached over with his left hand to unbuckle it, saying to himself, 'OK, the right hand is not working.'

'I remember even then just instructing myself: "Oh I can do this, I can get there."' It wasn't until his leg gave way and he was holding on to his wife 'for dear life' inside the entrance that the truth began to dawn.

During the first hours of confusion, as they were trying to establish the nature of the stroke, he started to 'run a film' in his head about his successful recovery. When they discovered a bleed, he was left reeling in a stroke ward, surrounded by the very ill: 'I kept on thinking, "What does that mean?" This huge cloud descended. This all felt very serious suddenly.'

He called out to a busy consultant who told him in passing that he wouldn't be out till next week. She then came back and 'interrogated' him about his drinking. 'I'd had a few glasses of wine the night before because I was upset about my cat dying.'

'I got so fed up, getting nothing out of these people about what was happening, that I decided all I could do to take control was to write.' Luckily, he is left handed. The lines he wrote set the tone for everything that happened subsequently: 'When I wake up I will feel my right side. I am going to get better.' And so on. 'It made me feel better.'

Finally, a compassionate consultant arrived ('He was visibly upset about my cat dying!') and explained what was going on. And during the night, on the hot, noisy, ward, he felt his right foot swivelling involuntarily. 'They were pleased about that. I looked around. There were some really sick people there, several with aphasia, one person who could only communicate by blinking... I began to count my blessings: I can see, I can speak, I can hear.'

He realised that he had a choice: to focus on either what he did have or what he did not have any more. 'That was a turning point.'

I ask him what gave him the ability to do this. As someone who has had mental health problems, I know that changing one's attitude is not something we can all do so readily.

David goes back to a story at a conference in 2007, where he heard a speaker, W Mitchell, share his story of recovery from a motorbike accident that left him with over 65% burns, who was also left paralysed after a plane crash! His mantra was: 'It is not what happens to you, it is what you do about it.' He also maintained that if you focus on good things, you will get good stuff back.

David, fortunately, was also in a position to feel that he could train his brain. He wanted to write his learning down and after a few weeks already started to think he could help others by doing so. 'I knew my mental state would have a profound effect on how to get through. And, practically, how can I ensure that I do this? So I decided to keep a diary.'

He shows me a diary entry from two days after the stroke: 'This still amazes me: "Getting the right mental maps, the language of recovery, how you approach the process of recovery from anything is critical, choose your words in the positive and with specific outcomes in mind, that way your feelings will be influenced hence your energy and strength, an example of this is 'I will walk again, I can see myself walking soon, I am so strong that nothing will stop me getting back to normal,' run films that show yourself getting back to normal, taking your first steps, lifting something, small steps..."'

When listening to this, what strikes me is the level of detail. That specific steps and long-term outcomes were part of his written drill. That it was not just about him, but also people around him. 'I saw this as a systemic thing, so it was people around me, family, friends: "We will be successful, it will be a breeze."' He pauses and laughs again, but he is clearly emotional reading this back: 'Well, obviously it wasn't a breeze! But it was about setting the intent.'

He is emotional because he knows now how close he was to dying or being left severely disabled. His consultant had confirmed this later, after acknowledging David's recovery as one of the most astonishing he had witnessed – so much so that they would want to learn from him. And his gratitude persists: 'These days, when I think, "I have not accomplished enough in my life or honoured the things I should have done," I switch to thinking that anything from now on is a bonus.'

There is a continuous theme of gratitude throughout the diary: 'I was so grateful that I was lunatic enough to think I could start working again. I was already thinking, "Well if I cannot walk again, I could still do phone work or operate with a headset" – this was on the first or second day of hospital!'

The quality of care and degree of compassion he received was exceptional. 'That first Saturday morning, I was sitting in shorts and a t-shirt, feeling horrid – I hadn't washed or shaved since being in the garden burying the cat. This male nurse, Andy, helped me to the toilet and then for a shower and shave.'

David remembers arriving back at his bedside chair feeling 'happy as Larry – if I can do these small things, it'll all be OK'.

More great care arrived, and then the graft and craft of recovery began.

'This incredible Jeanette, the physio, addressed my explosion of questions: "Why, when, how...?" She sat there, with great calmness: "The first two weeks are critical to engage with your physio. This is the time when a lot of movement can come back; you have to make time to engage and do the exercises. I will work with you and support you.'"

Once again, David noticed the measured and nuanced use of her language. He still remembers precisely what she said over ten years ago: 'I want you to take your affected hand (which was the unresponsive right fist) and I want you to take your left hand and I want you to open and close it and, as you do so, I want you to imagine your right hand opening and closing – visualise it, like a film, and keep at this. You won't notice anything…yet.'

David notes how that word 'yet' made all the difference – that it was a 'beautiful use of language – the strategic use of the word "yet"'. The physio explained how there would be little physical movement but a lot going on in the brain as it tried to reroute the neural pathways.

Small elements of communication mean so much to patients. And this is a message that still rings true for David and his work.

Little by little, his fingers began to flicker, and after two weeks he was able to open his whole hand. He was excited. Not just about the recovery, but also the learning and how it might be useful for others.

'This was also about my sanity. Because it was so horrible, I disassociated from it to some extent. I was able to take a kind of clinical stance, to establish a stance of curiosity. My intention became to have an awareness of what I was doing *for somebody else* in my position.'

He delves back. His mother was a chest physician – 'a model people's doctor with a wonderful bedside manner, a capacity and desire to listen to her patients – the shining example of great patient experience long before the phrase came out. I've always been interested in why people become doctors and aren't like that. Or don't have the capacity to be like that.'

David knows he was lucky to have exceptional care at Watford General Hospital. And he is specific about this: his cardiologist, Will, made an indelible first impression. He stood at the foot of David's bed, assessed the situation, read the notes and then said words that David would always remember: 'You're a young fit man; there is a very good chance of recovery. What I want you to do is forget everything – work, money. Just get better. Take three months out and rest. If you get better quicker than in three months, then it's a bonus.'

As David points out, 'The way he said it just gave me so much confidence.'

He goes on: 'This is where I want health professionals to get this. It is so important: how you walk into the room, how you present yourself is so key. If you have this body of expertise, if you have the intention to make this person better, then a patient must be able to *feel* that in everything you do and say.'

Though walking in the style of John Cleese in the Ministry of Funny Walks, he continued to work hard with the physios for his healing. Meanwhile, he was investigated for the causes of his bleed. The tests were always inconclusive. It was a one-off, they decided.

And he transferred analysis of his learning into a journal. He shows me page after page of neat, small writing in black ink. Deep insights, beyond mere aphorisms. He flicks through the pages, pauses at one particular early jotting and reads it out: 'I am recovering from a stroke which has taken out the whole right side of my body. The good news is that I am getting a lot of feeling back, however I am having to learn to walk again... I find the whole process fascinating and I guess this is what keeps me focused on the process of learning to walk again.'

The page shifts into a stream-of-consciousness set of affirmations, like 'Every movement however small mastered in a consistent way is a major victory, my equivalent of climbing Everest,' and then back into the broader learning: 'When I walk again I will look back at the magic of the physios and their marvellous skills of putting people's lives together. There is of course the whole mental strategy of piecing this whole thing together successfully of what I need to see, hear and feel at each stage. The key is to focus on the micro-steps, these important outcomes...the sound of footsteps. All this spoken via the internal voice congratulating me that this feels good, that this is valuable feedback. In this way I will see the difference.'

While David is reading this all out to me, my mind drifts to top leadership programmes in the NHS, ones from which patients are excluded. It strikes me, yet again, that these pages may pack more punch than most modules. And delivered with an integrity that many 'experts' are unable to draw upon.

But David's humility shakes me awake from such pompous dreams. 'This was an exciting journey. I could have looked at all this differently and focused on all the faculties I have lost. Instead, I tried to imagine what a stronger and more determined person I will be...and I kept on thinking about W Mitchell.'

It was not all positive, of course. He describes a frightening experience when, exceeding the physio's expectations, he was left loosely supported to take a few steps. This was when he became acutely aware of how self-talk could have toppled him: 'It was like standing on top of a mountain to ski. I kept on thinking I was going to fall, but somehow managed to shift to visualising the outcome I wanted and to a new commentary: "I want to make three steps, from here to there. I can do this. I can get there. I just move one foot. Then the other."'

He says he felt the old voice came with a wobbly feeling and the new voice effect a visceral change. And he stepped across the room. A huge milestone.

Not long afterwards, he had a vivid dream of being able to walk. He remembers this event so clearly. He had pinched himself in his sleep just to check that he was 'not dreaming' and woke up! Four days later, he took his first steps and walked on his own; his dream had become reality.

He had taken his journal right away and written this stream of consciousness: 'I am an awesome walker, I am a great walker, I love walking, it's a joy to walk again, walking the talk is breath-taking, I am walking my dream, I am my dream of being able to walk again, I can feel my walking legs, I love the sensation of walking, I can walk to the toilet yee-ha, dancing soon, I can feel my calf muscles strong again, I am walking my dream, I can walk to the stars.'

For many, this may sound odd, even slightly inane. But David explains that the power of the phrasing is that it is at 'the identity level', a phrase well known to communication experts.

'When you adopt something at an identity level, it can be very powerful. So, for example, if you say, "I am useless," that's probably the worst thing you could say to yourself. But if you say, "I am great," etc., that's the complete opposite.'

Yet still, while I am listening to David's account, something bugs me. He had left this seemingly successful work, well paid and full of international holidays. Why wasn't he at least a teeny-weeny bit resentful and negative? I sure as hell would be.

He explains that he had never thought like that. It just did not occur to him for whatever reason (though the fact that he had disliked his 'cold-calling' type roles may have softened the blow). Maybe it was also that a new career was already opening up, at least in theory.

His stroke consultant, also called David, wanted to learn from him in two ways. First, about how to support patients in the two critical weeks after a stroke when many people apparently 'give up' – how could patients take back some control of their own capabilities? Second, what professionals could do to improve the stroke recovery process. So, David was invited to talk to the medical team and share his writings in the spring of 2009.

The feedback was positive, with one clinician agreeing that much of the learning was generic and could apply to other physical conditions, such as cardiac illness and amputation recovery.

Here were high-quality health professionals yearning to listen and learn – wanting to work together to change how they did things: 'I was very excited, I began to call it my "stroke of luck"; it was opening up such fascinating opportunities. I was so pumped, and, as I talk about it, despite the frustrations that came later, there is still so much to share.'

While listening to David, I recall how when I was ill, I would fill my noisy head with affirmations that drifted into meaninglessness, how I could not make anything stick.

Apart from the difference between my head then (stuffed full of uncontrollable negativity and anxiety) and his, there is the fact that David was drilling into the detail, the specifics. As he says: 'I've got underneath the car with this.'

He developed a structured approach to teaching, breaking a day's event into three parts and a framework that included learning for patients and for professionals. The feedback astonished him, and while there was money in the system, the national networks set up to promote good stroke practice paid him a reasonable amount of money to come and work with them: 'They loved it. I was going somewhere.'

He was asked to speak at major events, with different sorts of professionals. He reads out proudly from a report following a University of Oxford international seminar on 'The Patient's Perspective on the Fundamentals of Care' in 2012: 'A highlight of the seminar was listening to David Festenstein's story of his own experience of recovering from a stroke. After all the thinking and debate of the day, David brought everything back to the real essence of high-quality care: to focus on the person in front of you.'

The talk was intended to be 20 minutes long; it went on for almost an hour. David was also interested in bringing about change in training and education, often asking his audience to imagine being in the patient's shoes, stepping into their world, hearing, feeling and seeing the world through their eyes, to know what it is really like to be that patient. He was starting to design more sophisticated ways of getting his message across.

One clinician's feedback at another talk that David gave said it all for him: 'I will never see a patient in the same way again.'

And then the money ran out. 'I ran into the "speak for nothing" or £100-a-day sort of thing, and it was not sustainable. I had to go back to my cold-calling.'

Now he looks back more dispassionately. 'I had this dream that I could take this stuff and make money out of it basically. I felt resentful when funding was withdrawn. There was a lot of restructuring, they brought together different networks for different disease areas and I couldn't get a look in.'

'I was sort of lost, so I spent inordinate amounts of time thinking that if I could get to the top people within the NHS they would in some way recognise the brilliance of this and it would be embraced in some programme.'

He spent a lot of his own money knocking on the doors of private sector organisations to ask whether he could adapt his teaching to promote wellbeing in the workplace. No luck. He went to the pharmaceutical industry. Just small pockets of work.

He met people who seemed to promise things. 'They said, "Oh yes, this is nirvana, this would help so many people, blah blah," and it just went nowhere. I don't feel I cracked the marketing side of it. How to position it away from the crowded market of "patient experience" where people get away with bringing in patient voices on the cheap.'

The final straw came when he was asked to speak at a huge NHS innovation event. But instead of being a plenary speaker on the 'glamorous, vast theatre stage in front of thousands, with cameras and sound equipment with professor this and professor that and minister blah blah', he was part of a so-called 'pop-up university' at the back of the hall: 'It was so obvious how hierarchical and them and us it all was. They had beautiful theatres for the likes of the high-ranking officials and seamless tech. Us patients were at the very back, in a cramped box, with flimsy cardboard surrounds, with a mic that did not work, the booming sound of the plenary drowning us out.'

He remembers one courageous audience member later speaking up at the front: 'I don't think much of this set up. This is all about innovation and patient experience. I don't see any of these big professors and health gurus mixing with patients. They're all mixing with themselves.' Again, David laughs.

We are now into discussing the barriers to patients being successful innovators more generally: 'It was just a self-aggrandisement thing.' David tells me of innovators who gave up on breakthrough surgical equipment to make a living in Silicon Valley.

And by now, David was fed up with nobody listening.

I ask him to think about the reasons for the NHS being unable or unwilling to take on board people like him and his sort of ideas. His major explanation is about the inability to listen: 'Sometimes, on reflection, I think I gave the talk, but was just there to give the talk, and I was not sure they were really listening. Did they really hear what I said? More sadly, is this going to affect anything that they do?'

I push him on this slightly superficial answer: 'In fairness to NHS bodies and those who work there, I think, and this is very strong language, but I think they are imprisoned in processes. Which don't allow them to entertain those types of insights. It is to do with a lack of time at an individual level perhaps. And a preoccupation with systems and processes at a more strategic level.'

'Maybe, through hectic processes and the emphasis on efficiency, we marginalise empathy. These NHS bodies who rattle on about integration, pathway redesign and the like, they use phrases like patient engagement but there doesn't seem to be much engagement. There is a lot of not listening.'

And, for a few minutes, we discuss our shared experiences – the insidious ways that NHS bodies eke out others' expertise. How the introductory conversation begins with an invitation to meet with somebody who is working on this or that project and 'loves' our work or presentation. How this appeals to the ego, then they send you a document to comment on, or an invitation to meet others, and you suddenly realise it is a whole day's work to do so. But you do it out of flattery and hope and passion for the cause. And, as David puts it, 'They come back afterwards and say, "We've only got 10p."' And expect us to be thankful.

David continues: 'The reason this irks so much is that I know that the top consultancies going in charge ridiculous sums. But we are not valued.'

But, being David, he refuses to dwell on the negative.

He talks about his wife's amazing support and the love and care he got from family and friends. And before we go to lunch, he shows me a journal entry written two weeks after his stroke.

It seems appropriate to quote this in full: 'I've now been in hospital for two weeks after a stroke which took out my right side. I appreciate being able just to get to the toilet, have a shower, etc. I have required an enormous amount of help. I must say the nurses and physios have been nothing short of outstanding. They have been my arms and legs over this period. At no time have I been made to feel like I was a nuisance or demanding in wanting to fulfil these basic needs. It's a tough brief. They come in at 8am and leave just before 8pm – a long haul, and I have been amazed by their humour, patience and above all their very caring approach.'

'Not so long ago I had facilitated a presentation on "personal brand". The importance of congruence was highlighted as you carry out your day-to-day role. The hardworking team of carers really did provide great models of this. One lady, Gail, who used to shower me in the morning, had done this for 32 years. She still had a lovely smile very early in the morning and always had a bubbly approach to her work. Pablo, who worked very long shifts and weekends, had a 1.5-hour journey each way to work and, on top of this, again, always had a lovely, caring way in all he did.'

'Lastly, Rita, the nutritional support worker, who just radiated wonderful care and compassion as well as masses of positive energy. I thought that the way in which she cared for her patients, including myself, was so exemplary that I later on recommended to the chief executive at the time that trainees and other members of staff could learn so much from her empathetic approach and ability to truly understand the patient's world and make them feel so much better.'

'I thought of Marshall Goldsmith at the Professional Speakers Conference in New York where he asked us to think about the time when we go to meet our maker, to review all our achievements. Would we be happy with what we had achieved? These people, I am sure they would be happy. All the people they had cared for, whose lives they had pieced back together, what a wonderful feeling it must be to have made such a contribution to so many lives – to each and every one of them, I say this experience has changed my life so much. I must learn to appreciate the beautiful things in life, not to take for granted the very basic gifts that God has given us, to be able to walk and talk here.'

'What can you take from this story? Well, ask yourself when you wake up, what can you be grateful for, what can I focus on, look at the physios – I think they are magicians, the way they look for and read signs in the body to see if there is any movement in the muscles. Piecing together so many lives.'

He puts the journal down. Visibly emotional.

So, what will he do now? David trained as a communications specialist, coach and professional speaker and wants to help and support people with significant changes in their lives. He once helped a lady who had not flown for 15 years because of a past incident get back on a plane and fly again. Another time, he helped a man who had been in the King's Cross Underground fire travel on the tube without having to relive the horrors of the event. He recalls still, with pride, being described by the chair at a medical conference as 'a great example of someone who had coached themselves to wellness'.

A few months ago, he landed a big contract in his new business development role. As we speak, this ends in a couple of weeks, and there is a crossroads ahead. He is also refreshing his coaching credentials and his dream seems to be Skype coaching. I ask him whether he has considered dipping his toe back in the healthcare waters, and he is cautious. He knows that what he has learned might help those 'on the road to recovery' but refuses, justifiably, to make too bold claims. And he is unsure that he has the energy to try and fail again.

But you never know. His daughters, who run a YouTube channel called 'The Festenstein Sisters', have been gently probing him on getting back on his healthcare feet and sharing his specialness. Perhaps someone reading this will give him a call.

BEING
BELIEVED

Patrick Ojeer

You start this journey with one simple aim. You just want a better service for those you love... The passion stays alive when you realise it matters also to others. And then to have a wider community of those who want the same thing – new friends and relationships. Those things are far more important than getting rich and status.

Being disbelieved was the beginning. Patrick was looking after his young son who had sickle cell disease. He did not think they were getting the right form of care and he seemed to be 'fighting with the hospital team and consultants. They weren't listening. Luckily, my son was transported to another hospital and into an intensive care unit [ICU] where they were much more understanding.'

The London-based consultant they met there helped

shape Patrick's sensitivity to the limitations of professional expertise: 'Dr Minou advised me to find my own way, as consultants are inculcated not to admit their uncertainties.'

The contrast between poor- and high-quality care was the spark for Patrick's patient leadership journey. Once in London, and witnessing the sort of listening and good relationships that good care entailed, things got better for his son. And, Dr Minou persuaded the original team to listen to what Patrick had to say: 'He told them to accept my expertise and do the best they could to do what I had suggested in the first place.'

Like many people affected by long-term conditions, Patrick felt he 'knew more than they did' in many respects. He had started keeping a daily diary with his son, and was noticing clues – how, when he caught a cold, an acute exacerbation of his condition would follow a week later. He told the school and ensured his son wore a hat, and the number of colds he suffered went down from eight to nine a year to two to three. 'After a while, I was actually raising other people's awareness knowledge, suggesting things. And things I suggested got done. I found that pleasing.'

From that moment, Patrick was regarded as one of the team. In fact, things developed so swiftly that some professionals assumed he had been medically trained. 'And, of course, for my son – he improved, got well and was discharged.'

For Patrick, who had grown up with an instinctive sense that people from all walks of life should be equal, it was the moment when he felt he could have influence. This was triggered by an awareness on three levels. First, he felt that if he could make such an impact with an individual powerful consultant, perhaps he could do that more widely in the system. Second, he began to think that if he could make a difference for one person, he could help others in similar situations. Third, he had witnessed a huge gap in provision.

He had the fuel injection of passion. But he was alone and had no plan. 'This seemed enormously big and I didn't have a clue! The best I could do was to try and influence better care in the best way I knew how. I was lucky. Because at the beginning of my journey I met Dr Mabel Alli, director of North West London Haemoglobinopathy Managed Clinical Network. Mabel was instrumental in helping me to utilise my knowledge and meeting my ambition.'

'She supported me also in representing the network and the newly formed All Party Parliamentary Group [APPG] for Haemoglobinopathy, and to be a patient representative on the NHS London Specialised Commissioning Group.'

Patrick became chair of a local support group that hosted meetings of people with similar conditions and invited professionals into those discussions so they could understand each other and work together. Like other patient leaders, he often felt frustrated with the slow process of change. He felt there were many vested interests that resisted improvement, particularly around the edges of health and wellbeing – issues like social care and housing.

It was only when his profile was raised – by giving speeches on gaps in care and compassion at regional events – that he became a member of a London-wide network and developed alliances with people affected by sickle cell disease and other long-term conditions. He began to see that the patient movement was effectively working in silos and needed to come together. However, he felt that things were shifting in a positive direction in service improvement.

'I tried to find out more from others who had experience.' But the resistance was still there. The professionals – both at an individual care level and at policy level – still felt that 'they knew best and "you cannot tell me anything", so no engagement. Full stop. Disaster.' At that point he was beginning to have reservations about the journey he had embarked upon: 'To be honest, I would not have joined had I known the implications and changes that would be brought about in my life.'

However, another hope for improvement came when he was invited to speak at the inauguration of the North West London Haemoglobinopathy Managed Clinical Network, the first network in England for sickle cell disease, set up in 2001 across different sectors: 'There was huge interest, representatives from all parts of care, nurses, consultants, social services, commissioners. I was invited to be a member of this network; I didn't understand it all. I thought I must make an impression and a difference.'

Being accepted and spreading the value of sickle cell care is a consistent theme for Patrick. Though a naturally confident human being, the power structures within healthcare have been a constant challenge and he has needed to draw on all his natural charm and personality to get where he has: 'I slowly began to feel like an equal. I contributed as best I could. I had to insist on certain things and be forceful, but I was clear and so it was accepted.'

The need for clarity, presence and good communication

skills is crucial, it seems. But patient leaders don't have the support networks that allow for 'professional' validation from peers. Or from professionals. A sense of vulnerability can haunt the work. 'This is where you judge yourself, because people don't tell you. It was only years afterwards actually that I felt more influential. And this was because I was invited to a London-wide network that focused on commissioning specialist services that included for sickle cell.' But that opportunity itself posed challenges.

For professionals interested in leadership or a more strategic role, this sort of 'step up' may feel like an obvious and desired thing. But Patrick was not sure at first: 'I resisted, as I didn't see it as a way forward. My son was doing well. Had I overstayed my welcome and effectiveness in these sorts of networks?'

'This was a fork in the road. Do I go back to my previous life or carry on the cause? It was tempting to go back to my career in engineering. I was looking for a way out! But this new life was really interesting. I could have had a really comfortable life! Why was I thinking of continuing this unpaid and undervalued nonsense?!'

'But it was dawning on me – what we are doing is immensely important. You see so many people struggling with such an awful disease – people crying when having a crisis. The consultants don't seem to understand how best to address these sorts of issues. It's really awful to witness that and it affects you greatly. It's that sort of experience that keeps you going. And I was lucky: I could try to help change things.'

Luckily, Dr Mabel Alli had some power, believed in him and his work and shared his passion, values and belief in people. Patrick laughs: 'She coerced and encouraged me to get involved in this strange new world of commissioning.'

It was a surprise to Patrick that someone in the system would take such an interest in his contribution. She would share draft reports, ask for his views at informal visits to cafes and take his views seriously. She got involved in a piece of work on standard setting and nominated him to represent the sector in the newly formed APPG on a parliamentary review of standards.

This was an important step up. He had gone from condition-specific work (sickle cell) to working in broader areas around long-term conditions. He had also gone from a local demographic area to thinking London-wide. This is pretty normal for clinical and managerial leaders, but for patient leaders' pathways to shift in this way is rare.

Mabel was hugely influential as a mentor and ally and kept him briefed and supported. He also had to develop other knowledge (largely in an unpaid capacity) in his spare time.

'She kept in the background. She died, sadly. Only in her passing did I realise what great things she had done in Africa. The last time I saw her, I drove her home and we had a fantastic conversation. I had not realised her worldwide impact, how she'd been in her previous roles at Unicef, the World Health Organization, etc. I thought, "Wow," and she was so, so humble.'

This was Patrick's first real taste of genuine collaboration – where those from different perspectives joined together for a common cause. He was particularly impressed by people with HIV. A common assumption is that people with one condition cannot look further than their own agendas. Patrick found this to be untrue: 'People with HIV were hugely influential, really nice people and had a broad outlook not only on HIV, but seemed to have more compassion with other conditions. They were so interested to know what was going on with people with sickle cell disease. I remember one said: "Oh yeah, I met quite a few people with sickle cell disease at a local London hospital and in so much pain. More ought to be done." I just felt that the penny dropped – for the group as a whole.'

It was soon after this that particular nationwide arrangements were put in place so that sickle cell services were commissioned more strategically and systematically. This is still a source of pride for Patrick. 'I felt I was making a difference.'

But it was also the process. 'I liked the group, the structures. I saw many commissioners committed to the cause. There were 31 local authorities; some, but by no means all, brought patients as representatives with them. We were beginning to have a real voice.'

Patrick believed that patients and carers had to be central also to changes in service – what the NHS calls 'reconfiguration'. These are contentious decisions at the best of times. And often these decisions are made behind closed doors, or consultation is done too late for fear of public reaction.

Patrick saw first hand the added value of having patients in the room. 'They often don't see the value we bring. It is about compassion and the human element of course. But it is wider than that. When patients have to travel a long way, access becomes a family matter. Any change is a disruption, and if someone has more than one condition, this becomes increasingly fraught. When you change a service, it is disruptive. Changes in relationships with people and services have to be considered.'

Patrick had been part of the Sickle Cell Society since his son was diagnosed. He helped identify a CEO in 2012 who could take the work the society was doing to the next level – both strategically and, most importantly, in how it could be more connected with patients and carers. He feels that the society has made great strides but is reluctant to accept any praise for that. His natural humility is palpable.

'I am quietly pleased with the platform I may have helped provide. Since then, the society has been better in many ways – financially, in its position in healthcare.'

But he is most proud of how far the sickle cell care has improved since he was first involved: 'People had struggled with their own illness; most were told they would not reach adulthood, so to look forward was difficult. Patients have had to rely on benefits and social help, so they haven't had the ability to be independent enough to contribute.'

A recent encounter with an advocate reminded him of how far things have changed too in healthcare, both in terms of service provision, but also in terms of people's influence in those changes: 'I was talking to a 60-year-old complaining about normal health problems. I commented, "You do realise that in an earlier era, you would not have reached 30?!"'

Over the last decade, Patrick has found himself on the national stage. He helped planning around the Health and Social Care Act of 2012 that (again) reshaped how commissioning was undertaken for specialised services (that now includes sickle cell disease). By now, he has mastered much of the art of negotiation, relationship building and influence that are critical in the patient leader's repertoire: 'Those interpersonal skills, tactics, push-pull, different tactics every session, engaging clinicians so that they could be reminded about what patients need and how best to get to that.' He adds ruefully: 'I am sometimes successful.'

He points out that though patients are usually in a formally weak position – lacking knowledge of how decisions are made, unsighted as to how budgets operate and blind to the cliques that actually hold power – they are sometimes free from formal accountabilities, so they are liberated to say the things that insiders may find uncomfortable.

But it is still about power: 'They don't give us too much – they are the experts, with the position, the culture of being in that hierarchy; they don't want to share that and don't want collaboration... People say that patients have personal agendas. Maybe, but when I look back, I see clearly that when you get to the so-called higher levels, the national agencies, for example, a lot of it is about individual agendas and self-interest, not about help in real terms.'

Patrick has been fortunate in being made aware of the Collaborative Leadership and Health Research Collaborative (CLAHRC) Northwest London. This was one of the first organisations to encourage patients to apply to be Improvement Fellows – a year-long leadership programme focused on quality improvement and collaborative leadership. This course augmented his natural curiosity and abilities, and he found another group that gave him a sense of belonging.

He also then undertook an MSc, during which he wrote a dissertation on the limitations of being a patient and public representative. As a CLAHRC Fellow, he also visited the respected US Institute for Healthcare Improvement (IHI).

He got a shock: 'They opened the doors to us, showed us the quality improvement methods and tools, amazing!' While he was in the US he attended a lecture at the Boston University Hospital. This was what was known as Schwartz Round, a particular form of reflection where practitioners would openly discuss a case. Coincidentally, it was about someone who died due to complications from sickle cell disease. 'I was astounded by the ignorance, which could affect my son and kids of many parents similar to me. I was cringing about comments from specialist nurses, how people with sickle cell disease were labelled as drug addicts – that they were always complaining, always in pain. I was so upset, I had to leave.'

The path to being a patient leader seems to be two steps forward, one step back (that may feel like ten): 'Yes. It's something I have come to terms with but haven't liked. In my previous life, I always had an aim and I'd achieve it. It's not easy to come to terms with the roller-coaster ride with no idea where it's going. Do I have a clearer aim? Do I know where I fit in? Do I get anything back?'

He leaves the questions unanswered.

And what about the skills required? 'Basically, I am still Patrick, a human being. You develop, you really find out your tactics, wherever there is a new set up, learning about every individual, listen as best you can, think where you feel you can influence, increase your knowledge.'

He describes how he is now broadening his reach. He has been impressed recently with an international event that brought patient leaders from around the world together with professionals: 'I was sitting on a table with people from Norway, Sweden, Canada, people helping to change how services are happening. I'm encouraged!'

'My journey began from a situation of desperation, a broken heart and a feeling of being crushed, but I was hopeful. I never gave up. At times I was in despair, as I underestimated how slow the process to bring about change was. I feel much better that the services for those with sickle cell disease have improved and are continuing, slowly, to improve.'

His continued optimism and confidence perhaps stem from his family life in Guyana, where he was brought up with self-confidence and a belief in his own independence, as well as an avid interest in politics and political personalities. 'We were up all night watching elections, and I was fascinated by good leaders, whatever their ideology.'

But, ultimately, it is his dogged pragmatism and opportunism that shine through. He is doing this work for little financial reward. And he regularly sees professionals he works with receiving much more credit and status.

'Like many patient leaders, money is not so important. Of course we need to pay the bills. Embarking on this journey of being a patient leader is the greatest uncertainty. It can bring a huge amount of stress. How are you going to pay the bills? You don't really dwell, because you have to move on, because there are so many other barriers.'

He then goes on to give one of the most complete reasons I have ever heard for doing this work: 'But, this is personal.

You start this journey with one simple aim. You just want a better service for those you love and those who are loved by someone else and people who have no one to support them. The passion stays alive when you realise it matters also to others. And it is a good and fulfilling life to try and do that. And then to have a wider community of those who want the same thing – new friends and relationships. Those things are far more important than getting rich and status.'

His down-to-earth nature seems to come from his professional experiences – as an engineer, but also from odd jobs done while caring for his son, like minicabbing: 'I basically like people and have always been interested in others, and have always built up my own networks.'

I ask him about how he manages his anger – a tricky one for many people. He surprises me: 'When I'm really emotional, connected to the work I do, I am far more alive, more powerful. This is not a weakness.' He adds: 'I don't take anything personally. There are nice and not-so-nice people. I don't feel intimidated. I just want what's best; there is no time to dwell.'

He says that talking for this book has also been valuable: 'We don't get enough opportunities as patient leaders to share with others. This is my passion. This allows me to feel good about myself, to talk with someone who understands.'

'It is of course exciting to realise you've achieved something but you don't dwell on it for too long.' However, his central source of pride remains personal, of course: 'I am sometimes pleased with what I have achieved. But then I look at my son developing into a young, independent man. That is what matters.'

And what next? 'The plan is always evolving. There is so much more to do. What you thought was a big impact turns out only to be one strand of something bigger.' The 'something bigger' might be the future of the NHS itself and how it deals with resource issues: 'We want meaningful collaboration so we can address the difficult issues, how to use resources to get maximum benefits in a time of austerity. We have to talk openly about limitations and restraints. These conversations are not happening with patients, carers and the public yet.'

Research is another re-emerging interest: 'I saw the hidden suffering of people – mainly black of course – who had sickle cell disease, and its impact on lives. And the disproportionate amount of money spent on other conditions. There is lots more needing to be done in research and it is not being taken seriously enough.'

'Looking ahead, I am hopeful that my son and many similar people with sickle cell disease will realise their full potential with improved care and services. But this won't happen easily. There is no time to dwell.' And then Patrick is gone – to his next meeting.

HEALTHMAKER

Karen Owen

As people with health conditions, we have had to be curious and questioning to survive and navigate the system. We know the little changes that make a big difference to our experiences of care and we bring an outsider perspective that helps challenge the status quo – our challenges help people in the NHS reflect on their perspectives and our skills help in their development. They need us.

Karen visited the 2012 Paralympics during a 'mid-life gap year' after a 23-year career in the pharmaceutical industry. What she witnessed changed her life – not so much the heady haul of British golds or array of sporting genius, but another sort of talent – the Games Makers. These passionate volunteers were everywhere. They kept the nation engaged with what was happening, supported people getting on to trains and into venues, managed queues and generally cheered everyone up.

'I kept on thinking – this is something we need for health... Everyone acknowledged them, they were well trained, clearly branded and there was a pride in their belonging to a community that was giving something back, making things better for everybody. They made all the difference, the glue between the cracks.'

The concept of HealthMakers was born. Or, perhaps, topped off. Because Karen had already been thinking about her own experiences of ill health. She has lived with a rare condition called hereditary angioedema (HAE), diagnosed at 15. HAE is a rare but potentially life-threatening inherited condition. HAE symptoms include episodes of oedema (swelling) in various body parts including the hands, feet, face and airway.

Karen suffered bouts of face and hand swelling in childhood and teens, had to take lots of time off school and was hospitalised three to four times a year with excruciating stomach pains from puberty onward. Later she suffered anaphylaxis (allergic shock) to fresh frozen plasma. In her early fifties, she suffered serious throat swelling. Fortunately, a new medicine combination gradually allowed her to better manage the condition.

The four principles that improved her own health were: peer support, self-management skills, helping others to live healthily and working with others to improve the healthcare system and to improve wellbeing in the community.

'The Expert Patients Programme helped reinforce my

self-management skills. I learned as much from the other participants as I did from the tutors. But after the six weeks we were left hanging.'

'A few of us kept in touch for a while, but then the energy dropped off. It is so hard to make those links and keep them alive. You need proper, organised peer support. When you connect with someone who understands the daily challenges or is in the same boat, it really helps. Because then you have other people who you can ask: "When I had this, I felt like this – is that what happens to you?", "How do you deal with...?" and "Have you experienced...?"'

This seemed to her different to having a conversation with a clinician who understands what should happen but may not understand what helps your quality of life – about getting out of bed in the morning, actually facing the world, the emotional side of living with ill health, not having the energy to get up and financial worries.

She understands how fortunate she is to have reasonable self-care skills, a good education and a support system. But whatever your circumstances, she thinks you can benefit from the sort of support she has had in order to gain control and quality in your life (whatever your health condition). Karen, who is passionate about singing and part of her local Glee Club UK choir, uses the language of 'civic engagement, walking, dancing, singing, being a member of the community'.

Her ability to look after herself grew exponentially with additional support from HAE UK (HAE UK supports people to better understand the condition and push for equal access to treatments across the country). 'They run an amazing

Facebook peer support group which is vital to my self-management.' She became an active member in this support group and attended HAE UK's patient conference. This involvement meant 'giving back, gaining more confidence and being provided with a wider support network'.

She joined Twitter and followed various people who were talking about the NHS and patient involvement who she could never have reached in the real world. After lurking for a few months, she got braver, making connections and adding the odd comment about her own struggles with life and living with a health condition.

This led to her attending a patient involvement workshop, where she met me and Anya de Iongh. 'I finally felt then I was part of a community, on the right path.'

She was asked to join, and then chair, her GP surgery's Patient Group but was struck by it having 'no rules, structure or objective, so its purpose was largely determined by the GP practice'.

She adds that the various labels and acronyms, such as PPG or PPE (Patient and Public Engagement), do nothing to help public understanding or encourage people to join. Nevertheless, she persevered, helping to create a network of local groups that gradually became recognised as bringing good ideas to the table of decision-makers (at this point, the local funders or commissioners of services were called primary care trusts (PCTs)).

The network developed a document based on the views of people from 15 practices. This document survived a major NHS restructuring in 2012 and was used by the new commissioner (the Clinical Commissioning Group or CCG) to help improve local services. Better still, Karen was encouraged by a local GP, Dr William Tong, to be on the local Bracknell and Ascot CCG Board (as what is called a 'PPI lay member').

Gradually, she learned the ropes, helping the CCG to be formed in the first place, supporting it to be better at communicating with the public and slowly challenging the culture of the organisation. This led to better involvement of patients and the public in commissioning (the planning, design and delivery of services).

All the while, she was getting braver – online and offline – and trying to get people to think differently about what people who had health conditions could contribute. National opportunities followed. She was asked to speak at a 'Digital Doctor Conference' alongside Dominic Stenning and others. There she witnessed true collaboration.

'I don't care whether we call it being a patient leader. It's the ethos. Being able to make a difference by using my skills and experience as an equal in the discussion.'

Twitter and big events are one thing. Real change is harder. Frustrations followed. 'There was no easy way to get involved across the system – little way to demonstrate the benefits of our expertise.' Meanwhile, the HealthMakers idea circled in her mind. 'I needed a simple framework to bring the ideas together. I started to find it when I looked back over my own experience to see how things could have made my journey easier.'

Since then, what Karen has achieved, in my opinion, is staggering. Locally, she managed to pioneer her Health-Maker vision by gaining the support of the CCG Board and finding the funding for a pilot project. She has overseen the emergence of a community of people who are supported to undertake the elements of the HealthMakers model:

- People improving their own health as:
  - self-managers: looking after themselves and managing their own conditions
  - peer supporters: receiving support and playing a more active role in helping each other.
- People contributing to healthcare as:
  - facilitators: volunteers contributing to community wellbeing by delivering self-management courses and attending events to spread the word about health, healthcare and patient and public involvement
  - patient partners: being part of collaborative involvement and participation to influence change in health services.

This model underpins everything that Karen believes in and is one of the clearest manifestations of patient leadership in the country.

It builds on the understanding that people need to be encouraged and supported to look after their own wellbeing and then provides a clear path for deeper involvement, as well as the training and support.

She brings out a diagram that she developed with a close friend and professional colleague, Michaela Tait, Patient Experience Manager at Milton Keynes University Hospital NHS Trust. And she carefully goes through it – her passion is obvious, and you can tell she is systematic, professional and totally committed.

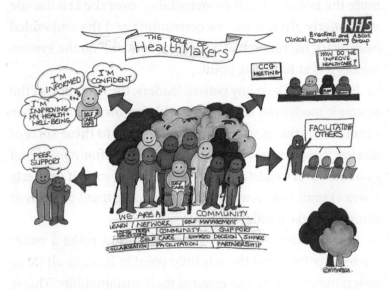

The role of HealthMakers

Pointing to the role of self-managers, she says she is keen to consider the way the NHS benefits, as well as individuals. 'If we only did this bit well, it would make a huge difference – fewer people coming into the service. In fact, this should be for everyone, not just those affected by long-term conditions. Unfortunately, not everyone can do this, because of our fragmented society.'

She returns to her views about inclusion of people from all walks of life throughout our interview. She is keen to declare that 'patient leadership' is about bringing all voices to bear. It is not an elitist sport.

Both Karen and I agree that there are many 'self-management' programmes out there. The NHS has tried to promote the notion of 'self-responsibility' over the last decade, particularly given resource constraints and the embedded healthcare narrative that 'excessive demand' on the system means it is at breaking point.

For Karen, like many patient leaders, the evolution of the strategic model ran side by side with her own story at a personal level – this is what provides the 'grit' to these sorts of stories: 'I always said I was good at looking after myself, but I was still overweight and did not look after myself properly. It wasn't until I believed in what I was doing that I prioritised things to make a difference.'

Karen points to her own experiences to make a wider strategic point – that there is little point in funding all these programmes unless one ensures their sustainability. This is why the other elements of her model are equally vital. Some people need peer support before being ready to consider self-management training, some need it to support them through the training and many will continue to dip in and out of peer support indefinitely. Much could also be provided by the voluntary sector and community groups or online.

Then, if people want to play a more active role in the community, they can themselves become the peer supporters and champions of the work. 'These are the facilitators, who have their light-bulb moment and want to give something back.'

Karen is trained as a volunteer facilitator and knows she has to 'walk the talk'. She set goals in the first HealthMakers self-management course she ran to lose 3 stone in weight and to investigate local support. She hit her target in exactly a year but is far prouder that four participants from that first group are still active HealthMakers.

People might then go on to become entrepreneurs, help to design an app for self-management or set up charities. They may work in GP surgeries to support wellbeing initiatives. Or they might go on to be involved in changing healthcare itself. This work is the cornerstone for collaboration, and though she has witnessed good work locally, she has powerful things to say about systemic barriers to this.

This might include shining a light on the darkest, perhaps least transparent area of healthcare – being someone who sits on a board, a committee or team meetings. In NHS parlance, this is 'governance' or 'scrutiny'. It is about holding people to account for what they do and ensuring oversight. This is where there is still precious little patient engagement.

Meanwhile, she has seen many attempts to provide professional leadership training across the NHS, few of which include patient leaders. When they do, they largely depend, she says, 'on the right people putting themselves forward or being identified by others in the know and it is often the same people there'.

However, the fatal flaw is to not value what patients bring. And from there, the consequences are massive. 'Many clinicians and managers want collaboration, or say they do. Many admit that it will help save resources too. But few seem to believe that good collaboration means that everyone – including patients – should be in the room. They say it, but they put so many barriers up to prevent it happening that it feels that they don't mean it.'

Karen calls on her professional background. 'I know how systems work and have been closely involved in programme budgeting, systems thinking and the like. Don't tell me I am "just" a patient – don't write me off like that! Even those without my skills can be trained and supported to do this.'

'As people with health conditions, we have had to be curious and questioning to survive and navigate the system. We know the little changes that make a big difference to our experiences of care and we bring an outsider perspective that helps challenge the status quo – our challenges help people in the NHS reflect on their perspectives and our skills help in their development. They need us.'

The clue to making this framework come alive is recognition that 'patient leaders', or, better for Karen, 'HealthMakers', should be recognised for the different things they can do: 'Despite being driven by its own grading and banding system for managing staff, the NHS likes to lump all patients together in their possible contribution. We are "consulted" or "involved" but rarely collaborate as equals. It is done in a way that health professionals would decry at an individual level, given their sophisticated diagnostic skills.'

Karen acknowledges she was in the right place at the right time, and that Bracknell and Ascot CCG was forward thinking. She was supported by GP director Dr Martin Kittel, who shared her passion for encouraging self-care and prevention.

In creating the pilot, they realised it was crucial for the training for the HealthMakers to be of a high standard. They chose Lynne Craven and Kerry Hepworth of the Self-Management Partnership for the self-management programme and Mark Doughty and me from the Centre for Patient Leadership to plan and define the initial training for patient partners.

However, the biggest barrier to the HealthMaker vision was how funding and commissioning works in the NHS. NHS organisations operate in silos and are as yet unable to bring all the elements of the HealthMakers model together properly.

Karen draws on her own experience as someone who has a rare condition to make the point about how commissioning does (or rather does not) work: 'These pathways for individual conditions are not straight-line pathways that everyone will jump on and walk the same way. We all have different things we bring to the system, that we all have to contend with, but what is not working is the link between the needs of people with less common conditions, like me, who need to connect to the "main pathways" at times (such as for my other physical health needs) or for those who cross paths in other ways (as for mental and physical health conditions).' However, commissioners usually purchase services via condition-specific (or what they now call 'programme') budgets.

I try to join up what Karen is saying. Would patient leaders who were truly involved in commissioning help? Would they be able to say at an early stage, 'Think of the connections,' between people with mental and physical health problems? Would they be able to ensure that providers who have the remit for treating people in a hospital are better linked with prevention and public health services? Karen nods. Simple. Not easy.

Karen hopes this will change as new commissioning approaches emerge. But: 'There may be a will, but I am still not sure the system's in place, either to commission services in the right connected way or to engage with patients and the public in the best way.'

Karen has a particular interest in data sharing in order to overcome some of the fragmentation she sees in healthcare systems. Her background in the pharmaceutical industry and project management, in addition to her patient experience, has revealed how critical this is. 'Nobody is making the real, brave, system decisions and supporting the real enablers (patients working together with staff on digital solutions).'

She fears the recent 'Care.data' fiasco has not helped at all. This was a clumsy top-down, non-inclusive NHS England approach to data sharing across systems, led by the former lead at NHS England, Tim Kelsey. The irony of this was that he also headed NHS England's work on patient and public engagement.

She is encouraged by the Berkshire Wide Connected Care Project for Integrated Health and Care Records. 'It has had significant patient and public involvement, even if it is not as diverse or far reaching as it should be,' she notes.

Karen is charitable about the seeming failures of central agencies when it comes to patient and public engagement. 'There are people in there trying to do good work, but they can't put their heads above the parapet.' She has also seen national and regional attempts at developing networks of 'lay people' fail.

This all has implications for the way in which any

network of patient leaders is developed – it needs to be truly patient led: 'The system is siloed and fragmented – when people get the need to be involved, the system puts barriers in the way, there is no integrity and it is tick box. The system doesn't provide a framework for true collaboration and partnership working.'

I ask her why that is. Her first response is to consider attitudes and behaviours of professional leaders – whether clinical, managerial or those in policy development: 'There are too many egos at the top. Health professionals who are pioneers of improvement work – many whom big themselves up on social media and are charismatic and personality driven. But they fail to include patients and the public or they do it too late. They say, "Here is my idea – now let's get people involved." That's not true collaboration.'

'Remember, many of those who shout about improvement the most at least have support – they get paid, they know the ropes, they are part of colleges, receive training, have career opportunities. Patient leaders have none of that – they have no choice; collaboration is the route by which they *have* to manifest leadership if they want to make change.'

She says a personality-driven leadership style may be endemic in the health system. 'It may be a case of "not invented here" syndrome. People become so invested in the need for recognition; they can become part of the problem.' I probe on why that may be the case and she softens slightly: 'Perhaps people don't feel acknowledged or valued enough. I know many who have just been battered one too many times by trying to do the right thing.'

I ask her whether she thinks patient leaders sometimes

have egos too! She laughs. 'Well, I see many banging the drum and advocating for one set of people over another. Or getting so angry that they can put others off and, ironically, prevent change. I think they need to get the other part of being a patient leader – that it's about an overall service. If it is not sustainable, it's not actually going to provide effective care.'

Karen is passionate about the NHS. She was and is happy with much of what she has received from clinical services. But she recognises deeply the pressure that frontline staff are under – and particularly the need to support non-clinical and administrative staff. 'I felt that administrators in the middle made my journey harder, due to poor systems. But I realise how people in those lowly positions, who can see how systems are not working, should be empowered to have a say.'

Karen could advocate for herself. Most cannot: 'I had to steer my own ship in a way that 80% of the population would not be able to. That is what I am fighting for. After all, if I get dementia in my old age, who is going to be fighting my fight?'

Throughout the interview, Karen interweaves her personal, professional and life knowledge: 'I have been in and out of A&E since I was five years old. Nothing makes me more upset than seeing a little old lady on her own. I have often got out of my bed to sit beside someone who is in total fear, with no blanket wrapped round them – staff with no space or time to help.'

I note that Karen has been using the word 'system' quite a lot throughout our conversation, and I am keen to unpick that a little bit. What has she learned from her unique vantage point as a patient leader involved in local commissioning of services – about how CCGs understand needs and plan and fund services? And, what helps and gets in the way of commissioners being champions for true patient and public engagement, as was the dream a decade ago?

Her response is stark: 'They just don't have the capacity to bring patients into the room. They have ridiculous timelines that everyone must work to and inflexible mechanisms of commissioning. They must meet assurance frameworks and this and that framework... It is just not possible to get the bums on the seats at the same time. This leads to so many tick-box exercises.'

I ask her for examples. 'We did a really great piece of work to develop an urgent care centre. Patients were included in the design and in deciding which provider would get the money to develop it. They helped ensure the brief was met and were at the table when critical decisions were made. And I am convinced that the service was absolutely different to how it would have been with sole input from managers and clinicians.'

I sense a 'but'. There is one: 'But I saw how hard it was to ensure true engagement, and it only happened because I am passionate and was able to spend the time to do it within a timescale that didn't work.'

Part of the work to be done then is for people like Karen to convince her colleagues of the value of patient leadership and patient/public engagement more generally. I wonder how successful she has been in this tough task. 'I am proud of what I have done. A GP colleague on the CCG board said to me recently, "I have you on my shoulder. I am constantly thinking – what would Karen ask in this situation? Have we got the right people round the table to decide on this?"'

We move towards discussing the personal costs of this work. And where is the balance to be drawn between challenge and being collaborative? 'It is a genuine dilemma. Part of the answer for me is to draw on different hats – my professional hat that comes with the skills I have acquired through doing system management and change control, understanding people the way I do. Then there's the life-experience hat from being a patient, being a mother, understanding the dynamics of my being educated and privileged. And then there is my "health-condition" expertise – different from going to the GP for a cold or needing to be fixed when you break something. A rare condition shines a particular light on a fragmented system and helps you point that out – sometimes in a helpful *and* challenging way.'

She emphasises her previous role – that it has provided her with a wide array of insight into complex systems like the NHS: 'I know about programme management, change control, how systems work together, the importance of data integrity, data quality, etc. Many around the NHS management control room just don't have those skills or experiences. I can help. If I can help, I make it safe. If it is safe, I can challenge. I can ask, "What if...?"'

But Karen, along the way, had lost her ability to wear these different hats. 'I had allowed myself to become labelled as "just" a patient. I want to remove "just" from all discussions! Unfortunately, my self-esteem took another massive hit when I was perceived to have a conflict of interest and forced to resign from my CCG lay member role in order to take up a support role with the local provider to continue to develop the HealthMakers work. Yet, I watched as other professionals seemed to straddle the two territories of commissioner and provider. I wonder whether patient leaders are being judged differently?' She lets the question hang in the air.

This latest knock-back came at a difficult time in her personal life and at the same time as a diagnosis of DCiS (ductal carcinoma in situ) breast cancer. However, she is coming through yet again: 'Support through trauma counselling has enabled me to see that I need to be kinder to myself. Self-management is a continuing task. Learning to love yourself really is the greatest love of all!'

She also sometimes sees herself as between, or even inside, opposing camps. As a lay member of a CCG, she was an outsider-inside. And she felt 'othered' by both CCG staff and some of the community and lay representatives on the outside of the system. But she has drawn on other sources of support, such as social media connections, friends, the ongoing peer support: 'There is a voice in the wilderness called Twitter. I see the value of working together in a way that the system itself has not done yet.'

Meanwhile, Karen still believes in the merits of having some sort of national network for patient leaders: 'I have not given up completely. I saw an attempt to do something like this, for lay members of CCGs, but it didn't really work. And I think that "lay" people who are not patients by experience fail to understand that we need a place to come together for ourselves. And what I saw with some people in national agencies suggests that we need to do it for ourselves. But I will not waste my time banging my head against a brick wall.'

And what are the chances of someone planning and supporting an area-wide HealthMakers programme with all the elements in place? She shakes her head. It is clearly not happening at the moment. She points out that one commissioner may support one bit, like self-management. Another may support another element, like peer support. And another – though this is rarer – a pool of patient partners or leaders who can help with improvement. 'Nobody is yet holding the ring. And nobody in the system yet believes in doing so.'

Karen has not lost sight of the vision: 'If you create this system of people who can look after themselves, they become your pool you can fish in. But you need to make it safe and inclusive for people to be part of it, create an ethos of trust. That comes from people within it being able to say, "Look, this is what it is like, let's work together to improve it."'

She and some of her colleagues have come to understand that the 'system' requires a multiplicity of patient leaders in different roles. 'After all, you don't say, "I need a doctor, any one of them will do," when you require cardiac surgery.'

This is where HealthMakers comes back into the frame. What if there were a large pool of people across the different aspects of the work? Who were ready, able, willing and supported to be true partners? At this point of the discussion, I am tired myself – the vision seems huge. It is something I have wanted to see for a decade at least. I stay tired, but Karen's passion rekindles something in me.

'I would love to look at some sort of "pathway of opportunities" for people.' I point out to her that I once had the notion of a 'skills escalator' for patient leaders – akin to that envisaged for nurses – so that opportunities and investment in opportunities and skills development went hand in hand.

She builds on this: 'There isn't currently an effective way to determine the different ways a person/patient/carer/ service user can contribute, nor to look at the competencies required to do so effectively.' She would like to see some sort of 'health passport' that acknowledges the experiences, insight and training someone gets throughout their health and care journey and covers participation in the four elements of HealthMakers. It could include those life skills acquired in life, volunteering, education and work.

This would allow for people's expertise to be truly valued and matched to the sorts of valuable roles in healthcare that should and could be made available in the healthcare system. People within an expanded HealthMakers community could then apply for the relevant roles – whether in research, improvement, training and education or governance.

I challenge her: 'But isn't this an "over-professionalisation" of what should be a more "outsider role"?' She replies, 'I am not stuck on labels. But you need a community that can be called upon, you still need the right person or people coming into the community because they need to – whether for self-management and peer support for their own benefit, or for the change work.'

She will battle away and now has a new role that means she can take the approach further. 'But I need to look after myself too. Know that my experience matters too. Then I am in a good place and happy that my small drop will be enough to create ripples.'

And we are back to the core of Karen's beliefs, based on decades of personal experience, professional wisdom and managing her condition and her patient leadership years: it is a tragedy that so much talent is wasted. 'This is not ego. It is written through me like Blackpool rock. Our wisdom has been wasted. You're not using those skills where you need them. It is like having a water tank and leaving the tap running.'

Many people in the NHS love a good framework and spout about a 'vision'. Fewer have the nous to make it real. Karen is different.

THE TACTICS OF INFILTRATION

Trevor Fernandes

This stuff is infectious – the people you meet, it's so different to the dog-eat-dog business world where you stand on people for fear of being weak. The people I meet doing this patient leadership work come from a different world – genuine people, unselfish, doing it because it's right, not for self-gain.

Trevor has booked a room in the august yet slightly austere premises of the British Cardiovascular Society. We are surrounded by oil paintings of robed male experts and glass cabinets displaying surgical artefacts through the ages.

Trevor had to book the room under the guise of it being for the society's business. I enjoy the analogy of the interview process – us as grateful-turned-surreptitious infiltrators.

Trevor has reason to be grateful.

He was a manager in a business environment with a good life. His was the archetypal fall. On 16 October 2006, his wife, Jackie, heard his agonal gasps – air escaping from his lungs as his heart stopped – and phoned 999. She tried to wake him and was told by the ambulance phone operator to pull all 14 stone of him out of bed. The bedside table went crashing onto the floor beside him as he fell. Everything was shutting down.

On instructions, she started pumping his chest desperately. Whilst he didn't return to consciousness at the time, that ten minutes got air through the lungs and kept his brain oxygenated. She saved his life.

Moments like that put everything in perspective. 'You can be the richest man in the world, but that accumulation of 25 years of working meant nothing.' But it wasn't over yet. He was given a year or two to live and told that the evidence suggested that only 8% of those with his combination of cardiac injury would survive.

He is still unsure why he proved the experts wrong and left them all scratching their heads. One year on from his heart attack, the doctors told him he had an 'ejection fraction' of 26% and diagnosed heart failure. However, this set him clear to manage the condition and live on; while not able to get back to his physical best, he would be able to contribute meaningfully in society.

All he knew then was his gratitude to the NHS. And his overpowering desire to give something back. 'I was being presented with an opportunity that I might never have had and I was going to grasp it, and do what I could.'

However, recounting the story now causes him to reflect

on the different phases of his 'journey' as a patient leader. His was a shift from outright gratitude and benevolence, through to bringing his own expertise – a combination of his experience with illness and his professional qualities – to the fore. This is the winning combination that the NHS ignores at its peril.

He decided to spend three years 'giving back'. It turned into a lifetime. The British Heart Foundation (BHF) asked him to meet people who had gone through his type of experience and offer them support. He was asked to give talks and be a representative for the BHF at various forums, and he gradually found his way into a policy advocacy role.

After three years, though, he was not ready to give up and retire. 'This stuff is infectious – the people you meet, it's so different to the dog-eat-dog business world where you stand on people for fear of being weak. The people I meet doing this patient leadership work come from a different world – genuine people, unselfish, doing it because it's right, not for self-gain.'

I joke that he makes it sound like he had been an ogre in his previous life. 'I was a good chap, but my business was quite ruthless. My former life was so different. It was a totally materialistic world. I got into bad lifestyle habits, didn't stop to think about anyone else. Now I see it all means nothing without your health. It's difficult to appreciate unless you've been through it yourself.'

Another blow came in late 2007. He had hoped that his former company, British Airways (BA), would offer him less stressful work. Indeed, he had gone back to BA to do talks to 'warn them what would happen if they didn't change their lifestyle... Sadly few probably could.' And he stayed friends with many of his former colleagues, who would visit and phone him each week.

However, BA forced him into retirement. A crushing blow. He felt cheated and had had no plans for retirement. The pressure on his marriage caused a temporary split. Trevor remembers grabbing the hoover from Jackie and saying, 'This is how you do it.'

'I was horrible – demanding control – but everyone said this was a normal part of the process and we just had to get through it. Devastated and worthless. I suppose some of it was ego. I had been the man in charge of a large department responsible for the BA IT network and now I'm a nobody. I was pretty depressed.'

Slowly, his frustration turned to constructive paths. He knew he had lots still to offer. He continued his BHF volunteering. And, at the end of 2007, Ashford and St Peter's Hospital asked Trevor to help set up a support group for people who use implantable cardioverter devices (ICDs). He built up a several-hundred-strong patient support group. He found the money to do this by taking on a piece of consultancy work in his former area of expertise – the aviation industry. He eschewed payment, but asked for his fee to be ploughed into the support group were his consultancy efforts successful. They were, and the support group suddenly had £10,000. This bought medical equipment too.

His two lives – professional and personal – had merged and he did this consciously from then on. At this time, too, avenues in the health policy world were opening up. He owes the BHF a lot. They gave him the 'in' to being a representative able to influence at Westminster during the period that led up to the Health and Social Care Act. The Act itself was to enshrine a corporate duty to involve patients and the public in ongoing decisions about healthcare changes. At a government health forum involving patients at Portcullis House, he found himself sharing a table with the then prime minister, David Cameron, and Stephen Dorrell MP, and banging his fist on the table when the ministers weren't listening.

But banging his fist and raising his voice have never really been Trevor's way. Tactical and considered, he carved out opportunities for influence. And it was his business sense that fuelled his perplexity about the NHS failing to value patients' views. 'I got involved in something called the NHS Future Forum. I saw an opportunity there. In the private sector, we have always consulted our customers about what they wanted and valued. I found it so alien that the NHS didn't do that. In that NHS Future Forum, we worked on the patient involvement duty, section 13H of the Health and Social Care Act 2012, which was intended to give effect to the policy of "no decision about me without me".'

Much of the patient-generated ideas at this forum found their way into Chapter 2 of the *Five Year Forward View*. (The *Five Year Forward View* was produced by NHS England in October 2014 under the leadership of Simon Stevens as a planning document.) The NHS constitution has always said it should engage with patients, but it was never enforced. 'Patient leaders like us can now go to the NHS and say it's against the law not to.'

Ever the strategist, he also knows that legislation is only

the first step. The next is to make it meaningful. During these endeavours, he noticed his motivations shifting: 'The reasoning changed; it became a crusade. I had this ability and training I had used in my job and could use that alongside my patient experience to really make a difference.' He has moved from 'gratitude and benevolence' through to the phase of 'Gosh, I can do this stuff' as a volunteer. Now his task is more conscious: 'It is about representing, equal challenge, due diligence. The NHS needs better scrutiny by taxpayers and the public – now I am also challenging from a public as well as patient perspective.'

It is striking that the nature of the role Trevor carved out is one that is akin to his former view of the world through a business development and operation lens – one that views improvement and change in the NHS as being dependent on the systematic use of levers that effect policy and practice change.

He talks a lot about making business cases – he tells the story of persuading a chief exec of a strategic health authority (prior to CCGs) that investing £100,000 in cardiac rehabilitation services (three specialist nurses and equipment) would avoid thousands of pounds in costs. 'It took over a year to persuade her – by showing evidence from national audits that only 18% of cardiac patients in the locality were offered cardiac rehab.' Consequently, readmissions in three to five years placed an unnecessary cost burden on the NHS and missed opportunities to save lives. He got his way.

This was in 2008, when Trevor and Jackie had moved from Surrey to Essex. He continued his endeavours to support local people with heart conditions and mirrored his former success to build another cardiac support group sponsored by Basildon Hospital.

While he was grateful to the NHS, he has never been one to wear rose-tinted glasses. 'I have a fear of not keeping proper records. We patients must always take our medical history with us. That's where things go wrong, where our care falls down a hole. The quality of care is dependent on the "handover" – from one GP to another when someone retires, from one consultant to another when you move home, from one health professional to another. The system relies on records and in trusting clinicians to look at them. It's getting better, for example in cancer care, but where the pathway crosses different conditions and groups of professionals, too often the system does not work so well.'

His international experience is another yardstick. 'When the ambulance comes, paramedics with iPads should soon have access to my full record. But in Scandinavia they've been doing this sort of thing for 20 years. In France, they have automated external defibrillators (AEDs) in all public places, and since the 1990s, they've had defibrillators in the lifts.' The frustration with implementation has become another passion.

His local and national work has steadily evolved. He is well versed in telling his story, and his eloquence won him and Jackie a five-minute TV slot to help raise awareness for a stem-cell campaign about 'mending a broken heart'. He organised an event at Writtle College, Chelmsford, to raise awareness of the research programme and raise funding by bringing all regional support groups together. And he networked and networked. On the back of previous work for the BHF, he got access to clinicians, professors and experts who came and helped make the event a roaring success.

His local, regional and national work was coming together. He got to know local councillors and policy makers, the 'stepping stones for what I needed to do'.

'My intention is always to start at the top at policy level, to be involved in every decision group down to delivery. That's the only way I can make change happen, because I would be the person to influence decisions. I put myself in as many NHS England policy working groups as I could, focusing on NHS commissioning and National Programmes of Care. For example, I joined the Complex and Invasive Cardiology Clinical Reference Group, one of 70 specialised services. This allowed me to influence cardiovascular services and have a voice in developing policy.'

His work in innovation reveals this staged tenacity. He knows Michael Seres well: 'People like Michael Seres have many barriers to overcome in getting their innovations adopted. We have so many bureaucratic hurdles and are lagging behind other countries in Europe. Surreptitiously, I used my presence at various bodies, such as the Accelerated Access Review and the NHS Innovation Accelerator, to influence the adoption and spread of lifesaving innovations, which were initially piloted in the East of England and were now being used nationally in the new care models. I like to think that I helped a bit to get low-cost, lifesaving technology used on the frontline, through the CCGs and Sustainable Transformational Partnerships. For example, the non-injectable connecter, PneuX, a system that prevents ventilator-associated pneumonia, and myCOPD, an app for better managing chronic obstructive pulmonary disease [COPD].'

This rigour is based on an assumption – one that traditional policy makers and health professionals see as on the wane in a more complex and fractured healthcare system – that policy and practice flow from each other in a pretty straightforward way. It is refreshing to hear a patient leader still somehow having faith in this centralised approach to decision-making. It is even more refreshing to find someone who has the tenacity and willpower to influence it from a patient perspective. He nods when I use the word 'infiltration' for what he does – for what we all must do. 'Infiltration is the path to better outcomes.'

At regional and national level, Trevor seems indefatigable. He has worked on innovation policy – being part of initiatives that ensure good ideas are not blocked by the wayward risk-averse regulatory structures that are deeply embedded in the NHS.

And Trevor knows he is fortunate to have that capacity and capability. Indeed, his main worry about the patient leadership movement is how difficult it is for some to manage their energy. His main advice for those who are setting out is to make sure they marshal their efforts as wisely as possible. As the demand for patient leadership inevitably increases, so it is crucial that people choose wisely – that they put their efforts into opportunities that will provide them with value and will make a difference.

Another special ingredient is love and support. From resuscitation to recovery through to his resurrected career, it is emotional support that has been the constant. When ill, he had recorded his experience in what he called a 'web of care' document. This depicted chronological events and the people involved at every stage and what they did.

It evidenced the importance of loving care from partners, family and friends. 'When I looked in detail at what people did for me, without a doubt I would not be here if it wasn't for them.' This web of care and emotional support is often intangible and is undervalued. There is little 'evidence' for the importance of love. 'You don't realise how powerful it is... It's about emotional support.'

For Trevor, this is about his wife, who 'put her life on hold', sisters, friends and former colleagues: 'My wife and I experienced some difficulties at first in adjusting to changes – this impacted our relationship, partly caused by the uncertainty and fear of what the future would hold... Thankfully, we needn't have worried too much. Simply, my wife is the reason for my survival and continued recovery. She resuscitated me at my time of need and then continued to care for me throughout my illness. She was my source of comfort and the voice of reason at a time when I could not make sense of anything. She was my link with the doctors and the outside world and she made all those difficult decisions on my behalf that have put me firmly on the road to recovery. It must have been so difficult for her. I had the doctors and nurses; she had nobody, yet she was there throughout, always with a smile and offering words of encouragement. She gave me the strength, confidence and purpose and she continues to do so. I am very lucky and I am concerned for those who don't have the loving support I had. How do they cope?'

Emotional and practical support is a common thread: 'It's about the basics such as the lift to the shops and the basic knowledge that someone cares. And, when the system frustrates you, it's about having that "care coordinator". I can give you so many examples – the frustration with miscommunication between the heart failure nurse in primary care and the consultant. I used to pull my hair out and my wife would say, "Calm down, I will sort it out." It took a lot out of her.' It almost goes without saying that patient and carer leaders need this unpaid role acknowledged and rewarded in some way. People who do this work are usually patients with long-term conditions themselves, and the emotional labour is immense.

And this is his latest crusade – after the gratitude for the NHS and technical side of care; after the building of policy and involvement in implementation; after the development of strong networks and voice, his return is to the emotional: 'Heart docs fix you, but they don't understand the serious need for psychological support. These is no provision for that. Nurses don't do that effectively, and if they do it, it is not part of the remit – they go on to the next patient.'

Given his interest in governance and scrutiny, it was perhaps inevitable that he would get involved in inspection and regulation. He was one of the 'experts by experience' in the widely respected Keogh Review in 2013 that experimented with a different model for inspection. The methodology was trialled in three hospitals, and Bruce Keogh himself, the leader of the Review, praised the input of people like Trevor as the 'most important aspect' of the work. This included creating safe spaces for whistle-blowers and community insight events where residents came to give views to the experts by experience, who they seemed to trust more than 'professional' inspectors.

He continues to divide his time between local work (on a Patient Participation Group), regional involvement (as chair of the East of England Citizens' Senate and within his sustainability and transformation plan (STP)) and national work.

However, Trevor looks ahead at the patient leadership challenge and is worried. He knows he is fortunate enough to be able to afford to do the work he has come to love. This is in terms of both his financial stability and his health, though on both counts he now has to be careful. And he and his wife have consciously sacrificed their former lifestyle for the work.

He points out carefully that patient leaders can't do their work if they don't have the means and that the only way to release them from work or benefits is if you can pay to release them. The NHS does not recognise this. He has seen this clearly. 'If you have a group of 50 people who are motivated – half of them will not be well enough to continue. They are inspirational but inevitably inconsistent. Of the ones left, perhaps half will have to work or have dependants, so they can't give themselves free of charge, so you're left with around ten people. If, on top of that, the focus of their energies is not useful, they are involved in meaningless feedback work or stuff that does not influence decision-making – at the top table, if you can call it that – then we have wasted everybody's time, energy and wellbeing.' He sums up the policy implications: 'I see opportunities that slip through our fingers.'

But patient leaders themselves 'have to be cleverer at what we spend time on. If we put a value on our time and what we donate, it's a huge amount. When I was working, my company charged clients £1300/day for my consultancy work. If you tot up how much we donate free of charge, it is a huge amount. We must not underestimate the value we bring.'

There is a lack of value given to this work, he points out. And that needs to change: 'I say to people, "I don't have an 'ology' in what we do. All we have is our experience and it is so important we learn from it. Whatever you do, make absolutely sure that it is focused and meaningful, think carefully about what you could do, as there is so much demand."'

One twist in this tale is that he has noticed that the patient voice can carry more weight than that of the staff. It may be because patient involvement is still a tick box and system leaders give way. But, as Trevor points out, if we are clever, this is a useful fact to remember. He also sees some progress in how the NHS accepts patient leadership. He talks about the NHS Leadership Academy and, in particular, the Nye Bevan Programme, designed to help organisations take their senior executives to the highest level of leadership. 'Our role as patients/carers is to ensure candidate responses are deeply patient focused but also that the programme is designed in a patient-centric way. So whilst I have reservations about leadership in the NHS, I can't help but applaud the efforts being made to develop the right type of leadership.'

He is also involved in a programme to build an improvement culture in hospital trust board members: 'It is very interesting, and my role is to scrutinise the programme design and challenge – which I do in abundance. So, once again, I applaud the leadership for implementing these programmes; they have a desire to improve the management ethos. I often feel the NHS can do more to improve services and quality of care, but they need to adopt the improvement culture and discipline often found in the private sector. We have been doing this for the last 30 years! In the airline environment, when a system works well, that's when there is potential to break it down and improve it. We couldn't afford to stand still, or else the competition would get the jump on us. So now I see it happening in the NHS – oh well, better late than never!'

So where to next? As well as being drawn to the issue of emotional support, he is intrigued by the quality of management and leadership in the NHS. He doesn't always like what he sees. He wants to challenge how managers do things and whether they are up to their job: 'It is public money, after all.' Managers and senior leaders must be accountable, and with this comes scrutiny.

He is not, though, as harsh as his messages perhaps convey. He comes back time and time again to the connections between people and has nothing but praise for the patient leaders he has met along the way: 'I got to like and trust people who do this work and hopefully I have become a bit like them. I hope I have changed.'

Reference

Keogh, B. (2013) *Review into the Quality of Care and Treatment Provided by 14 Hospital Trusts in England: Overview Report*. London: NHS.

TOUGH WORK

Lesley Preece

For me, the agenda is about continuity and integration and not falling through the gaps between institutions, silos and professionals – working with patients to have a say, not putting unnecessary barriers in the way of good healthcare. I do not want to take potshots or take out particular irritations; I feel I am contributing in a much broader sense. The work of a patient leader, or whatever you want to call it, is not for the faint-hearted or for quick wins. It is much more important than that. The changes we make could and should be sustainable and make a big difference to a lot of people.

It had been a difficult few months. Lesley was a headteacher of a school for children with challenging behaviours and learning disabilities and mother to five children. As 2004 drew to a close, there was mounting pressure.

She had led huge cultural changes that meant bullying (by staff and pupils) was on the way out. But she had been running a deficit budget and was fighting for proper funding to keep pupils and staff safe.

It was a difficult job to do at the best of times – Lesley has never been afraid to tackle the hardest of challenges. She tells wonderful, yet painful, anecdotes about the pupils and their parents – several dads belonged to local gangs and would sometimes threaten pupils and staff. But: 'We had the best cross-country team in the county because the kids were so used to running away.'

Meanwhile, two critical incidents occurred: no-win-no-fee law firms were leafleting the poorest areas and encouraging families to sue for non-events. And a father threatened Lesley and the deputy with death and was subsequently imprisoned. He'd been bomb-making in his back garden.

Both these incidents garnered press publicity, raised safeguarding issues and brought about local political pressure and staff and pupil stress. Lesley had to carry the weight of all this on her shoulders. In hindsight, an accident was waiting to happen.

One drizzly Thursday evening in January, Lesley parked her car behind the school: 'I was dying to go to the loo. I stepped out of the car, slipped, pivoted round and skidded under the back of the car. I heard a crack.'

Even from a hospital bed a few hours later, she tried to hold things together. The school was applying for 'specialist' status and concomitant funding and she asked her colleague to pick her up the next morning. Wishful thinking.

Lesley had dislocated her ankle and broken her leg. On

Friday morning, she went for surgery. All should have been routine.

'When I came to, I was aware of something pulling across my neck. I tried to say something and I couldn't. I was used to managing panic because of confrontations with children and parents. But I wasn't in control.' A ventilator was doing the breathing for her. And she was quickly put under again.

The operation had gone horribly wrong and she was lucky to be alive. A lump in her throat had prevented her from being fully anaesthetised, but also prevented withdrawal of the anaesthetic. And her throat had collapsed. Fortunately, an ear, nose and throat (ENT) surgeon in an adjacent theatre had performed an emergency tracheotomy – the only way of providing an open airway.

She woke up in intensive care with a 3.5-inch cut across her throat, unable to communicate, exhausted and surrounded by confused discussions and phone calls about being transferred to the specialist hospital (Addenbrooke's). Meanwhile, her tracheostomy tube shifted and she was left gasping for air. A consultant arrived from Cambridge with the wrong equipment for an internal evaluation. Finally, staff decided to leave her in Bury St Edmunds for follow-up surgery on the Monday (a biopsy of the throat lump and the leg operation).

Then her head swelled up: 'I felt a bubbling under my jaw line, like when you strain to blow up a balloon.' She was developing post-operative subcutaneous emphysema – too much air inside you that finds the path of least resistance. 'Over the week my head became huge. The bubbles were down to my elbows and way below my bust. My eyelids felt like bubble-pack. I was losing motor control and full of air with a queue of curious doctors who wanted to feel my unusual head problem for training purposes.'

More operations followed: 'It was awful. Anything that could go wrong, did go wrong. I had a dreadful coughing fit one morning over which I had no control. They sedated me but I was super-alert. I subsequently lost the ability to relax into sleep. I was exhausted but wide awake. I was very aware of everything…hundreds of heated discussions across me about how best to treat the tracheostomy wound.'

Lesley was, unwittingly, learning about holistic care, or lack of it.

'An on-call ENT doctor was called across from Addenbrooke's one evening. He arrived in a temper wearing a fleece and smelling of curry and cigarettes. He undid the stitches that were holding things in place and told us all that my shallow breathing problems were due to me making too much fuss.'

Having just about settled in with a team of staff she trusted, the next weekend she was sent to Addenbrooke's. She asked not to go: 'They bullied me, saying how I had a duty to myself and to my family, how I wasn't well enough to be on a general ward, and a lot of other stuff, some of which was true and some not. They transferred me on a stormy Friday night across the A14 during rush hour.'

The worst moment came when she was left alone in a 'barn of a place…shuttered high windows, like a loading bay in IKEA'.

That night was 'the most horrible yet…isolated from the world'. She was left with her dressing oozing, without tissues to wipe it, constipated and with no commode. The loo was 20 yards away, and putting her weight down on her sticks opened the cut in her neck: 'I saw my swollen head in the mirror for the first time and was appalled. Twice I called for help but nobody came. On the third occasion, they were terribly dismissive. I needed to know if my face would ever settle back in place.'

No risk assessment of the new setting had been undertaken. 'This is really important. I was expected just to get on with the next chapter of being a patient in a completely different environment – begging for help when I could get someone to listen.'

Eventually, she asked to see the senior duty nurse, who listened and took things in hand. And a doctor cut off the dressing and taught the nurses how to massage Lesley's head to ease the swelling and how to get the air out of the wound. 'I've seen a child with hydrocephalus, but there, the features tend to be spread across the face, but my face was tiny in the middle of this massively swollen head.'

These traumatic incidents were 'flashback' moments for her developing PTSD. And she had terrible dreams about previous incidents at the school. Mental and physical health problems are intertwined. She hallucinated while pumped full of anaesthetics. 'Your mind frees itself to go to places that are beyond your experience.' At one stage, she asked a doctor whether people in her position sometimes just give up. 'It seemed the easiest thing to do. She said that they often do. I felt integrity in her response – she had listened and taken me seriously. I needed that.'

With hindsight, she can clearly see issues of consistency

of care (for mental and physical health) across what the NHS likes to call a 'pathway'. These included issues:

- across departments and services within a hospital – she saw gaps when wards were closed at weekends and/or she was shunted between them or between general wards and the intensive therapy unit (ITU)
- between general and specialist hospitals – where she heard nurses making agitated calls and saw doctors having to do the 'horse-trading' to get access to specialist beds and, of course, the physical transition issues (including lack of risk assessments and being 'dumped' in a strange place, then being 'returned in a taxi wearing only a nightdress and dressing gown, bursting with subcutaneous emphysema')
- during the return home – 'Being left with an appointment for six weeks' time and a sick note stating I had a broken ankle that ended the day of that appointment.' Being left also to negotiate all the 'life' problems that don't go away when you are sick. They just 'become so much more difficult to avoid, manage or negotiate'.

And, at each stage of that 'journey', she witnessed the best and the worst of the NHS – fantastic staff struggling to cope with cumbersome systems, individual care that was second to none, but also fears of 'doing the wrong thing' in emergency situations and defensive practice – 'Some of them no doubt thought that I would sue them' – and some held other assumptions and prejudices, such as 'the nurse who kept referring to me in a derogatory way as "the headmistress"'.

From this she learned about vulnerability and power. About how difficult it was to offer constructive feedback: 'When the ITU outreach nurse counsellor visited me in ENT I asked if anything could be done about ITU risk assessments being repeated after transfer. She listened but said that they had little influence over what Addenbrooke's did and that although she would pass my concern on, I would probably have to take the matter up with Addenbrooke's as a formal complaint. I felt I had taken such a beating; I had no energy for that.'

And, beyond this, she kept on thinking about others who would be even less able to make their case: 'It's hard to be dismissed. When the stitches had been prematurely removed from the tracheostomy wound, I was continually concerned about who was coordinating my recovery. Physios had been instructed to get me up and using crutches, but when I put pressure onto the crutches the neck wound was forced open. Physios dismissed my concern and left ITU without talking to ward staff about this. Even though throughout my career I had battled successfully for safe provision for vulnerable children, I learned that you may not know how to make a fuss on your own behalf. It may be extremely difficult to judge how ill you are if being "ill" is not in your experience, and you may make a real hash of trying to stand up for yourself – you don't have the vocabulary or the grammar.'

Some years later, on being transferred from one ENT unit to another for the lump in her throat that had grown and become infected, the receiving clinicians paid no attention to the letter that came with her from her previous consultant: 'It said – please would they consult him. They didn't.' Lesley put on weight during subsequent years and at one time had a series of appointments cancelled at the last minute. She overheard herself being described by an acronym, 'SFWMIU', and was told sheepishly by nurses that it meant 'stupid fat woman making it up'. 'But I knew I had to get my file from the "too difficult" stack to the "quite interesting" pile.'

Listening to all this, I find it hard to know how Lesley now operates so professionally and patiently when she works with clinicians and staff as a patient leader. There seems little bitterness: 'I learnt such a hard lesson. I'd had very good support at West Suffolk Hospital, but then everyone knew what had happened to me, my file was flagged up, there was a huge amount of concern at the time and I was cared for. But how you transfer knowledge and information about your condition from one hospital to another – I had no idea how difficult that was.'

Lesley's previous professional career – indeed her whole family life and previous experiences with a large family – signalled the perennial need for respectful dialogue – adult-to-adult conversations about difficult subjects. This was one reason why she was later attracted to the notions of patient leadership.

But before that, there were mountains to climb. There were many things she could not do any more. Sleeplessness led her tramping around the house in the middle of the night to avoid waking her husband. She could not swim because of the cast and open throat wound. Nor could she sew, as she could not see what she was doing. Concentration in order to read and write was impossible (her spelling and grammar had gone).

'These were the skills of my trade! I had lost lots of grey cells but hoped they would recover. Eventually it became apparent that "recovery" isn't like getting back on a bicycle and pedalling off. It's much more like learning a foreign language or a musical instrument where you have to practise, practise, practise. In fact, I prefer "rebuilding" to the phrase "recovery". Even then, a weakness will remain and show up when you are under pressure.'

As she talks, I worry that the process of telling me all this is too much: 'Well, I'm OK. My emotions are running fairly high, I'm swearing and I'm frequently disordering words.'

She was upset about not having been able to hand over her head teaching responsibility properly – there is that 'continuity' issue again. 'The staff wouldn't let me have my diary so as to say, "This needs to be done, that does not..." This really mattered to me for a very long time.'

And her sense of powerlessness was almost crushing. It was partly to do with acknowledging that she wasn't going to be going back: 'I wanted to be allowed to step back with support.' Naively perhaps, she tried to go back to the school and finish the 'specialist' school funding application.

She wasn't getting far with her GP either, who 'treated me like any teacher with bog-standard "normal stress". But soon I was under mental health services and diagnosed with PTSD, and it would take several years to gain some sort of equilibrium.' Meanwhile, the school had not filled out the requisite accident forms so she (as the breadwinner at that time) had no money coming in. The drugs she was put on didn't help, and the stress was putting her marriage under pressure.

'I was also dealing with grumpy GPs and ENT, ITU, mental health, fractures and visual difficulties staff, as well as having no physio. Some in the education field suggested I was malingering. I was dealing with 15 silos in total plus friends and family. I now believe that if someone had been acting as an advocate, "key worker" or coordinator for me, those messages would have been so much clearer. I felt terribly alone throughout this time and really believe that if I had been entitled to recognised support, holistic medicine and an annual review, lots of things that have subsequently happened could have been avoided.'

She received an ineffective form of treatment for the PTSD and erroneous assumptions were made by a private 'trauma therapist' who said she seemed afraid of dying. 'The one thing that this all clarified for me was that I was not afraid of death but of being completely dependent upon somebody else. I had seen this in some of my previous pupils. Brilliant brains locked into completely uncompromising bodies.'

Eventually, she applied for ill-health retirement. But what would she do? Stripped of professional identity, full of high-level strategic expertise and experience, but lacking income, purpose or meaning. Despairing of the way the health system was controlling her, she discharged herself and tried to go back to studying a doctorate and going on a counselling course. It was too early.

She was the one who needed help, though, and eventually found a wonderful psychotherapist called Sally. Together, in

2006, they inched their way forward. But what should she do about her anger about the experiences she had suffered? One route was a formal complaint or even litigation. She decided against that. An NHS 'trauma' psychologist told her that would slow her recovery. This seemed good psychological advice, but at no time was she offered an apology – the system buffered itself from admitting fault or identifying learning.

While listening, it strikes me that Lesley has always had to 'hold things together': for her family while she was a young mum in the New Territories of Hong Kong – 'We were the only European family for miles'; when returning to England with growing kids and double unemployment; and in her 50s when her husband and she agreed she should become the breadwinner. The pattern continued into the hardest of jobs. Always coordinating, always at the hub of people's complex needs. 'I've always seen myself as a sort of quartermaster mother, making sure everything was in place, so that my children, who are so different, had the support around them to go off and do their very different things.'

Meanwhile, she had looked at joining a patient support group. 'But mostly it was about really angry people seeking to blame, and that wasn't what I wanted to do. I wanted to help make small changes that would prevent people from having the experience that I just had.' She needed an opportunity to share insights and expertise from her professional life in order to help others. Her career had meant improving leadership and staff culture, working with damaged children as human beings, maintaining effective multidisciplinary teamworking in severely stressful times.

The NHS, with its raft of self-help groups, feedback surveys and focus groups, did not fit the bill: 'In a previous post, I'd been head of education, with 112 pupils, 82 of whom were wheelchair users, one third with terminal conditions, working with physios, nurses, night staff, 45 teaching assistants... Recently, I'd changed a bullying culture...and the NHS wants to "involve" me by getting feedback? I could do that, but I could do more. That's not good enough.'

'I want to promote justice, information that is accessible, explanations and communication with those who find things difficult. I want to deal with equity issues – because I know there is always someone left behind.'

She turned to more practical ways of giving back and wrote a document, *Tough Work* – a guide for employers and workplace colleagues supporting an ITU survivor to return to work. 'If I could prevent some other poor sod from going through what had happened to me, there would be some sense.'

'But I learnt that hospitals and NHS provision don't have the capacity to respond to improvement projects from individuals – no matter how good and useful they might be. A second guide, *Tough Work Too*, aimed at supporting folk attempting to return to work with mental health issues, remains unfinished.'

Lesley also worked with an Indian paediatrician friend with mental health problems on a *Feeling Fine* recipe book with Indian and equivalent English versions of basic, healthy comfort food and a not-for-profit enterprise for protecting the intellectual copyright of bright ideas from people with mental health difficulties who were temporarily unable to develop those ideas. But neither project came to fruition because, 'ironically, neither of us had the capacity to take them forward'. She also dreamed of starting a small consultancy to support headteachers needing an independent critical friend, 'Two Heads are better than...', and good-quality documentation, 'Unfinished Business'.

And all this was when Lesley was at 'rock-bottom with self-esteem, lacking energy to break into established or unrecognised markets whilst keeping a roof over my head. Mostly, I learned that it is extremely difficult to provide for yourself whilst your sleep is trashed, your head is scrambled and a psychiatrist says you've misplaced your personality [the formal diagnosis that Lesley had been given was "enduring personality change after catastrophic experiences"]... So, I looked for paid work.'

Her first attempt – still with throat problems, atypical sleep apnoea and drugs she couldn't tolerate – was a project with a local charity that was supporting people with work problems due to anxiety and depression. 'Usually I was the first person who had the time and interest to listen to the complexity of a client's situation. There were big holes in the services to which I needed to signpost.'

After divorce, she took what she calls a 'gap year' to try and heal, walk her dog daily through the Brecklands in Norfolk and became a local Parish Clerk ('Think *Vicar of Dibley* meets *Monarch of the Glen*'). But when her elderly parents hit their 90s, she took a job near them in Hampshire as a residential retirement estate manager. Once again, she saw the lack of continuity of care, this time when one moves from the purview of one hospital trust to another: 'There seems to be no follow-through, despite letters a patient may provide inviting contact.'

In 2014, Lesley moved to Brighton and used the musculo-skeletal (MSK) services there. And there were still problems: 'I thought that I was retiring to Brighton to earn back my health. It turns out life doesn't work that way. You find that the various battles you have had to fight result in different bits of you ending up in different services with nobody looking at the whole. Then you are told by your GP that "you seem to be a very heavy NHS user". And the GP prickles when you gently tell her that actually the Industrial Injuries Disablement Benefit occupational health physician has the most holistic understanding of your needs because he understands that mental and physical conditions are part of a complex whole.'

During this time, improvements were being made to the MSK service to try and make it more 'integrated' and, after one of Lesley's family members got more involved in local patient engagement work, Lesley and I met. She wanted a purpose and became intrigued by the model of patient partnership that the local service was developing.

'From a series of gentle email exchanges with the patient director and a similarly kind telephone conversation, I learned that patient partnership at MSK was quite different from anything I had come across before. I was invited to a forum but got impossibly lost in and around Crawley and made the most conspicuous of entrances. I would have run away if David had not spent time giving me choices about how I could proceed.'

At the time, I was seeking to develop a pool of strategic patient leaders to get involved in projects to improve care and be equal partners in decision-making (see the last chapter of this book, 'Outsider-Inside').

Despite our service trying to make things more integrated, Lesley still felt she was being caught between different parts of the system. She had an ankle problem that affected her hips and gait, and she knew that she needed to be treated holistically, with decent physiotherapy and pain management – which is what our service has been trying to do. She had developed arthritis of the hips and had gained six stone since 2005 from not being able to move about, and all this was affecting her mental state.

During her time as one of eight patient partners, she has been involved in several projects working with clinical and non-clinical staff. She has worked with me on a project that has improved the way frontline admin staff deal with people who use our services, helping to design training for call handlers and changing the role descriptions of receptionists. Her passion for accessibility has recently led to her leading a project on improving how the service provides information and explanations for people who have particular communication needs.

Lesley has ongoing complicated medical issues. 'But being part of the group has given me a purpose and distraction from the rest of the rubbish in my life.'

Things have not got much easier. 'I've lost several imagined futures. It can be hard, but the more you dwell on loss, the harder it becomes. However, what actually exhausts me is always trying to strap on the armour of optimism so that you can face the day. You run out of the energy.'

So, there are constant different sorts of balances to be struck: between pushing passionately for change and managing one's own energy (tiredness, frustration, being triggered, loss of confidence); between utilising one's expertise and coming against systemic barriers to engagement (staff not having the time to engage, the speed at which daily NHS life happens). These balances are not understood or widely acknowledged by clinical and managerial leaders, who can either come to ignore outsider learning or see it as a free gift – of little value.

'I was at the top of my game when the accident happened and had a lot of skills, having worked my way from the bottom of the system.' But it's a slow process to come through and reapply those skills. 'Until this work with you, David, I have not been able to find a way of testing which of those skills I still have and then find a purpose for them. So that's incredibly important to me.'

Lesley sees the work we do around patient leadership in Sussex as unique. 'I don't want to be a fighting advocate for a particular patient group on behalf of one set of people over another. That is not my agenda. I remember regular meetings from hell when I was a county education advisor with advocacy groups being highly critical. I would always ask, "Who is speaking for the children who don't have a label?", and there'd be this silence. I want rich conversations, nuanced, it's the complex stuff I enjoy!'

Our work in Sussex attempts to bring staff and patients together and to model reflective dialogue. It is not about being 'driven' by one's own story but more about how people – staff and patients – reflect on their own experiences so as to help reframe problems and find solutions. One crucial part of Lesley's recent work has been to help me see how, instead of only using the patient partners for institutional projects, we can also gear things around what the patient partners want to do. This has led to one of the priorities at this time being continuity of care.

'For me, the agenda is about continuity and integration and not falling through the gaps between institutions, silos and professionals – working with patients to have a say, not putting unnecessary barriers in the way of good healthcare. I do not want to take potshots or take out particular irritations; I feel I am contributing in a much broader sense. The work of a patient leader, or whatever you want to call it, is not for the faint-hearted or for quick wins. It is much more important than that. The changes we make could and should be sustainable and make a big difference to a lot of people.'

This way of working is a subtle, but profound, change in how engagement is usually undertaken in the NHS. I often use Lesley as a sounding board and informal mentor, as I identify with her sense of sometimes being an 'outsider-inside'.

As we close the discussion, I start to wonder who is looking after Lesley. She pauses and laughs. Another story from her past: 'Well, me I suppose. When I was a head teacher, an Ofsted inspector asked me: "Where is the anger in this school? Unless you're holding it?" He was an interesting guy.'

Lesley now knows, through bitter experience, of the need for care and feels that the writing of this book is helping to provide space for reflection and support. But it is Sally, in Suffolk, friends and her family that she turns to: 'My kids are amazing. They are very, very interesting people. They have a lot of fun. They are properly busy in their own lives.'

She describes the discussion for this book chapter as a 'gift'. I say that I want to do justice to her story. She replies:

'Don't think about it that way. I am not expecting a therapist. I now need a way of bringing my skills to help change things.'

More pragmatically, Lesley is now more aware of circumstances that are too close to the bone, too resonant, too triggering. Those in the engagement world need to take this on board too. 'I think you are made very wary by your own healthcare experiences. You do have to learn how to retreat and protect yourself early in order not to "crash and burn". Not to drive yourself mad by agonising over the glaringly obvious gaps.'

Her curious and rebuilding mind may well take her towards a doctorate or some form of high-level study or leadership programme. But I am unwilling to let someone of Lesley's talents and courage go somewhere else too soon! I quip that the 'revolution' is in too much of its infancy locally for her to quit just yet!

But Lesley is coming to the stage where the notion of 'revolution' is not so much about the struggle. 'I am quite tired of "fighting".' We talk about the book's title. 'Revolution to me is the never-ending circle I've been around in the last 13–14 years. Let's call it a spiral. Sometimes up; but downward spirals are very grim.'

She tells one final story of a young Chinese teacher she knew in Hong Kong, who observed that Europeans see progress as a rolling forward momentum. But her view was of continually trying to keep things in balance – in equilibrium. 'That understanding has been really useful as I learn about what dynamic change means – it is not always about a driving forward... Spirals.' She smiles. 'Spirals.'

THE AMAZING FALL FROM GRACE

Ceinwen Giles

I have got to the point where I know I have expertise to offer. The system does not yet respect patient leaders... We are modelling a different sort of service provision – setting up the market stall outside the citadel.

When I meet Ceinwen, she is training for a triathlon: 'A small one,' she laughs. 'Well, I needed a hobby. OK, I push myself, my husband tells me to chill out – that I have a laser-like focus.'

Is that motivation from her experience of healthcare? 'Maybe, but it's been there before. Don't know where I got that from, maybe driven by fear of failure, like most of us.' More practically, it was her early international development work that gave her a glimpse into the world of suffering before she was ill herself.

After a bachelor's degree in geography, Ceinwen taught

English in Thailand, where she became fascinated by housing policy and intrigued by slums – their design and how people supported each other: 'We denigrate people, calling them "slum dwellers". It does not represent who they are.'

In 2001, at 26, she moved to Vietnam with a non-governmental organisation (NGO) to work on housing and social justice. She followed that with time in Bangkok and then in Sierra Leone soon after the civil war. 'I saw some terrible things, heard awful stories. And that was quite hard. I learned to put up some necessary personal boundaries. But perhaps crucially, it taught me that bad things happen to good people, for no reason.'

This was to help her later, when counsellors seemed to want her to work through the stock 'Why me?' and feelings of anger or guilt. She never had these sorts of feelings.

Ceinwen now runs Shine Cancer Support with her colleague Emma Willis. And the catalyst for that? Her illness. 'I was interested in whether yoga was available for cancer patients. It turned out to be yoga in a chair – the assumption was that chairs were needed because the programme was designed for much older people. I was 34 and thought, "Is this what I have to do now?!"'

She was put in touch with Emma, who was then running an informal group for younger people with cancer in Poole. After chatting over coffee, the two of them decided to work together: 'And we went blah blah we could do this, we could do that, all this stuff.'

Ceinwen's story is much to do with partnerships: 'As a consultant in the NGO world, I always advised organisations to collaborate.' I ask her about the tendency for some patient leaders to want to be superheroes and fix everything them-selves. She replies: 'It's very easy to let your ego think that. It wasn't going to work for me, and that has been the best thing. It is so hard to work by yourself.'

'At Shine, we are in charge, which is nice, but you can take ideas from others or yourself and run with them, rather than having 15 people to sign it off.' She is obviously fortunate to have struck lucky with someone she trusts: 'I work with nice people, but I do stuff that I can see makes a difference. That's where the energy comes from.'

She pauses: 'Over and above everything though, it is that I have personally been through the experience of cancer and its consequences. That's what truly makes the difference.'

We start to delve. In 2009, two days after a 34-week preg-nancy check, she was told her baby was too small and that she had to stay in hospital. Two days later, after terrible chest pain, her baby had to be delivered by caesarean. The doctors thought at first that Ceinwen had pre-eclampsia, and perhaps also 'HELLP' syndrome, a rare and life-threatening condition.

Her baby was transferred to a neonatal intensive care unit (NICU). After a few days of terrible sickness, Ceinwen was allowed home. But she still wasn't well, was on lots of different painkillers and was struggling with the baby. Af-ter a few trips to A&E, where she was told she should be in hospital ('I didn't want to be there, I wanted to be with my daughter'), she had to endure five long months in hospital.

At first, they did not know what was wrong and she was put on a liver ward, during a winter bed crisis. Surrounded by women with alcohol problems and one who also had dementia, it was 'a real eye opener. I was 35 and hadn't been with sick people in a hospital before.'

To make matters worse, she got lost in the system. 'Nobody came to see me for a couple of days, they seemed not to know where I was.' She eventually had some placenta removed and felt a bit better (in hindsight, this was probably due to her anaemia being helped by the transfusion during the operation). But, again, hope turned to frustration. And worse – the 'amazing fall from grace' as she puts it.

After a series of CT and MRI scans, as well as lots of other blood tests and X-rays, she was told she had lesions on her liver. A biopsy on a lump under her arm confirmed non-Hodgkin lymphoma.

In this whirlwind from wellness to ill health, the precise chronology of what happened remains, unsurprisingly, unclear in her mind. 'To go from being pregnant and out one night for a pizza with my husband to everything falling apart within a day or two.'

'I was by myself when I was told I had lymphoma, and I remember saying, "Oh, isn't that cancer?" I'd been in the hospital for weeks wondering what was wrong with me. I remember saying, "Right, this is bullshit." I got dressed for the first time in at least a week and went to the desk and demanded to see the consultant, because I thought they'd made a mistake.'

The consultant came the next day and told Ceinwen and her husband that it was stage four non-Hodgkin lymphoma ('the worst') and that she had to start treatment right away. 'I remember saying – you always hear this – "Am I going to lose my hair?" And then, "Am I going to die?"'

'It was the worst moment in my life. And it came so soon after being a new mum. I am not a big freaker-outer, but I thought I was definitely going to die.' The isolation ('At one point, I had to be put in a side room, as I was upsetting other patients'), and the stress of not being with her family, took its inevitable toll.

Months of in-patient care followed, while her husband looked after their new daughter. Even then, she noticed what was going on around her: 'You become institutional-ised and restricted in what you are able to do.' She saw this in staff too, noticing both the quality of care and the nature of interactions.

In particular, she remembers a specialist nurse who found out her dad was Welsh and began to teach her Welsh: 'He'd bring a new word for the day. It kept my mind busy while I was stuck in this isolation room.' But she also learned that these relationships run counter to professional bound-aries. She wanted to keep in touch with him when she left, and he gave her his number, but told her she must not tell anyone. 'I can understand a little why this is the case. But aren't they human beings too? They take care of patients for five months and then never see them again. They don't know if we have lived or died. That must be really hard.'

Those months were a hard time. 'This wasn't my plan for life; being in hospital was awful, sure. But I had worked with people whose arms had been chopped off... If that could happen to them – well, I'd had a privileged life.'

After months of chemotherapy, low on energy, with a high chance of relapse and all the while 'still thinking I was going to die', she went back to work three days a week. But then disaster struck again. She caught meningitis, as the drugs had wiped out her immune system, and was back in the same hospital again.

'Meningitis was the straw that broke the camel's back. Any kind of emotional resilience had gone. That was when I began to think, "OK, why am I the sick person?" You always think it will be someone else. I couldn't walk properly and lost 20 pounds. My daughter was 18 months old and I was away from her again. I was distraught.'

Throughout these periods, her boss was unsympathetic: 'That really shocked me, because I always assumed that if you worked hard, then that spoke for itself, and it doesn't.' She needed money, so she hatched an exit plan. And she was also mining her own experiences. Could they be useful?

'You spend six to seven months in hospital, you see so much that could be changed and I thought, "Why not try?"' Like many patients who want to get 'involved' she was funnelled into traditional patient and public involvement groups. Her previous experience showed her immediately that this wouldn't work. 'Having worked in community development, I wondered how they thought they could understand patients without understanding the communities they come from.'

She continues: 'I used to do work with women in Sierra Leone. The number one rule: don't hold the meeting when women are busy! Maybe early evening when they've come back from the field. I could never get over the fact that most patient involvement work is done during the day, then they complain it's the "same old suspects", and of course: it's 2pm on a Thursday!'

But it is not just about methodologies, she says; it goes deeper: 'Lack of power and the reluctance of professionals and institutions to let it go, paucity of skills and lack of training, organisations that don't allow for innovation or uncertainty.'

She tried volunteering in a new cancer centre, which she also found dispiriting. 'The main thing about this experience was that I really saw how the NHS has its own language, which is pretty impenetrable to outsiders. As patients, we were invited to meetings and given information but I didn't understand half of what they were saying – and in any case it mostly felt like we were being kept informed of what was happening rather than being given a chance to influence things before they happened. I kept on thinking, "There must be another way of doing things."'

Ceinwen applied for a Clore Fellowship in Social Leadership, a prestigious programme that provided bursaries, training, mentoring and coaching to leaders in the social sector. 'It completely changed my life. I was back on the up; quitting my job to do something different was such a good feeling.'

The turning point had come about for two reasons. First, Ceinwen wanted to put her professional expertise into action. Second, the healthcare experience had revealed a gap in services for people at her stage of life with cancer. She wanted to apply the principles of community development to supporting young adults with cancer.

This was also the period during which Ceinwen and I met. She undertook a feasibility study on the Centre for Patient Leadership as part of the fellowship and linked up with other 'patient leaders' beyond the cancer field.

After meeting Emma, who was running a support group in Dorset, Ceinwen's business brain kicked in and they brought the idea to London.

The work was pitched to people in their 20s, 30s and 40s. There was some support available for teens and those up to 24 years old, and for those over 65. Ceinwen loved the approach that Emma took with the support group. 'Emma went to cafes and bars, they did beach walks. It was really informal. Nobody had to go to a hospital basement, sit in a circle and eat rubbish sandwiches.'

Her husband, Steve (an epidemiologist by trade), suggested they do some research on the gap in needs and develop the evidence base. They did an online survey and got 244 responses within a couple of weeks. 'It was amazing. We knew nobody. We didn't have anything. We had a hunch. But suddenly we had the stats to show there was a clear need.'

They held a workshop to discuss the research and run their thoughts by other young adults with cancer. 'People didn't want to leave at the end of the day. We should have organised drinks!' Emma and Ceinwen knew they were on to something.

They then held a 'launch event' for the research with other people working in the healthcare field. 'People asked how much this all cost – I think it was £400 for printing and room hire; we did the event for very little and the research was done by me, for free. But it was very successful. People just got it immediately, could understand what we were doing.'

Emma, who was diagnosed with breast cancer when she was 29, was then still working as a bank manager, and they were both doing the research in their spare time. They held a second event at a Macmillan Cancer Support conference, but they wanted to develop things gradually. Informal meetings run by volunteers slowly grew in number, and the Clore Fellowship helped develop their plans.

'It has grown organically, with lots of different volunteers starting networks in their own places. We have 14 now.'

I say she makes it sound easy! 'It hasn't been, but we've been surprised. We didn't go into this thinking we were going to run an organisation that's going to employ others.' I interrupt again to ask where the idealism was. 'I did think it was important and did want to change the world; we just didn't have a sense of exactly what we would do and how we would do it.' It reminds me of a phrase that patient partner Lesley Preece has used: 'busking with purpose'.

Emma took redundancy from work and had a little more time. They had had an idea to run a retreat for younger adults with cancer. By 2014, a year after starting the Clore Fellowship, they were ready, with £5000 in the bank, ongoing forays into the crowdfunding world and Shine registered as a charity. And at the last minute they got money from the Big Lottery Fund and Macmillan Cancer Support.

They called it 'The Great Escape', 2.5 days for 23 people. It was successful beyond their dreams and is now an annual fixture.

So, what has she learned about growing an organisation like this? 'The personal experience is key. It gives you an insight into the issues that the people you support have, and they understand you, they trust you more if they know that you've gone through it.'

But I am also struck by how she seems to have put her ego aside. 'People have told us that they appreciate us not situating ourselves as experts. We try to think that we are all in this together – the community element is really important. That's what's helped us grow. Others have gone on to fundraise or tell people about us. We have grown on goodwill, not a lot of money but a lot of volunteers.'

She says the policy and campaigning will have to come later. They are at maximum capacity, and again she is stressing the balance between pragmatism and idealism. 'But it's mainly about the power of peer support, because I was missing it. I thought when I was ill, "Am I the only one that this has ever happened to?" So, I see how it benefits other people but I also see how it benefits me. I think that's still really core to whatever we do. And we wouldn't change that.'

During our conversation, at the back of my mind I keep wondering why the NHS can't see the power of peer support. Or perhaps it does, but does not know how to do it properly. 'The NHS doesn't recognise the value enough. That it can help patients have a better understanding of their condition, decrease isolation, provide that sense that what you are going through is normal if you are ill.'

Peer support is more than just a hand to hold. It is about clinical quality. She tells a story that brings it home. When she was going to an immunotherapy clinic every month, though the quality of nursing care was good, the language the professionals were using created a care gap. 'You hear staff seek to reassure patients by saying, "This therapy is well tolerated." But what does this mean? I am sure the pharma companies talk like that, but I felt like shit sometimes. And other patients did too. Patients are the ones who say, "Yeah I know, I feel terrible as well, I go home and I sleep or I find the therapy makes me feel a weird mix of nauseous and hungry." But to be told it is "well tolerated" makes you feel something is wrong with you, so you can trust patients and get insight from them that the staff don't have.'

Ceinwen feels that we have gone too far down the road of an 'industrial model' of healthcare and professionals have become institutionalised themselves at times. 'Professionals don't have the time. I am not sure how well they are treated, they are probably not paid particularly well, probably over-worked, tired – why would you treat people well when you are exhausted?'

Like others, she feels that it is time to bring patient-experience and staff-experience work together – that patient and public engagement and staff engagement are two sides of the same coin.

And this brings us back to the energy needed to do this work at all. And, like for staff, how to bring yourself to the work, particularly as it is the experiences that fuel the passion. How can you balance the passion and the need to maintain sufficient emotional boundaries to be effective?

Those who choose to re-enter the healthcare world will face reminders of loss and suffering every day: 'We lost a great volunteer and good friend last year, and someone on the last retreat had stage four cancer. I had a really tough couple of months where I thought, "This is just so much loss, so sad." And it's unfair – a lot of really good people who have a lot to offer, it's just unfair.'

'When you do this sort of work, you have to build up a

wall. I'm talking to you and tapping into things I usually don't. I know so many good people through Shine who are in terrible places, and if I thought about that all the time I would be a wreck!'

For patient leaders, without the institutional protection and collegiate ways of working, it may be even harder to turn off than it is for staff. Is there also guilt if one is not working to change the world all the time? Don't you need a rest? 'Emma and I have talked about this a lot. It helps to have a partner. I fear turning into a sociopath, without empathy, because when you're constantly dealing with hard things, you do need to keep it at a distance. As a leader, you have to maintain a little emotional distance at times. I love what I do, but sometimes I need a break from cancer. I try to have "cancer-free weekends" – not check my phone or Facebook. Then you see something in the newspaper... There is always something in the paper!'

On a personal level, peer support still helps. Ceinwen still has friends from the times she was ill, and she also keeps fit through running. And patient leaders are still patients! 'Remember, being a patient is exhausting. A nurse once asked me, "Is it really exhausting?" As if I was making it up. It really is. Managing your appointments, when those appointments are constantly changed or are in the middle of the day. Especially, if you have multiple things wrong with you, and you don't have anyone who takes a look at all of those things together, so you're the one who has to do it.'

Back in the professional sphere, one of the counsellors Ceinwen works with had sage advice: 'You have to have a story you can tell without falling apart. So when people ask about Shine, you can tell it without falling apart, so it doesn't tap into the deepest parts of it.'

It also helps that Ceinwen has some control over the work she does and the direction of Shine. Many patient leaders' work is mediated still through others: 'We're in charge. So we can decide our direction.'

The Shine approach is predicated on 'normalising' people's sense of being human and taking away some of the institutionalisation that arises from being trapped within a medical model. This can be challenging for health professionals too. 'We take people to the pub, and if they want a drink, they have one! Some healthcare professionals have questioned whether we are encouraging people to drink. We are not forcing people to drink – we're just saying that normal people go to the pub, so why not be a normal person, have an apple juice while you're there?! I don't care.'

Shine's approach is a practical antidote to the institutionalisation of healthcare that she sees. She talks about how we treat old people and the fight to keep people alive at all costs, regardless of quality of life, about nursing homes where people are not allowed to stand up because they might fall over and that 'the one thing that gives you humanity is being able to stand up to go to the toilet on your own'.

Shine also offers time and space 'to understand what's wrong with you, time to meet other people, time to discuss things – we try to take time to get to know people'.

This whole-person approach seems not to be possible within a system of silo working: 'Something has gone wrong with the way we think healthcare can be delivered. It's an industrial thing – your leg is broken, so we can treat your leg, or you've got blood cancer so we can treat your blood, but you can't deal with the depression because you've broken your leg and not left the house for six weeks and not talked to anybody – there's no holistic care in the system.'

And the added value of patients being able to point out these limitations seems obvious to her: 'Someone asked me once why it was important to have patients involved. It's because they can tell you how the system works, not how the system is supposed to work.'

She is trenchant about the limitations of the current traditional approaches to patient and public engagement. 'It's always about patients coming in to a system that is not working. It's not about the system changing. You can't just tag patients on to a system that's broken and expect things to change.' Like other patient leaders, she does less of the traditional engagement work: 'Some of the involvement I've had with the larger NHS bodies has not been very rewarding because they run out of time to do things properly or don't have the training to do it properly.'

'So you hear it with sustainability and transformation plans [STPs] – we want to involve patients but we are on a really tight time schedule, so we will do XYZ and then involve them. What does that tell you? That's not a commitment. The number of times I've been sent things late and they say, "We really want to involve patients, but can you do this by Tuesday?"'

There is a paradox here. People in systems think they should be the ones 'doing the involving' and at the same time fail to appreciate that working with communities is a very skilled job: 'In healthcare, we have the idea that anyone can do it. Oh, just go out and get some patients and talk to them, but nobody ever thinks about why patients should come and talk to you. Why should I give up my time to come into some crappy building at 2pm on a Wednesday where you get a bad cup of coffee? It's not a nice experience. Give people nice food, give them a thank you, give them a present – something to say thank you for donating your time. I find there's a lot of take, take, take and not a lot of giving back.'

Ceinwen is also easing back on her consultancy commitments, partly because the work is not understood properly: 'I ran a consultancy project with cancer patients in London, and the very first event we had with the client, they said it was the most diverse event they had ever run. But that's because I busted my ass going to the gay men's prostate cancer group, the Asian women's breast cancer group. I spent my Sunday afternoon in a gay men's group and they were lovely and I had a great time. And because I had made an effort to get to know them, then they were like, "OK, I will go to your event." The larger organisation didn't appreciate that, I don't think. They still thought it was easy.'

And what does the future hold for Shine? Ceinwen and Emma have a sense that getting to ten staff members will be a useful foundation (they have four at the time of writing). They have 24 volunteers who coordinate their Shine Networks, mainly clustered in the South, though they do have networks in Manchester and Newcastle.

As the charity expands, Ceinwen is aware of different sorts of challenges. She is well aware of 'founder syndrome': 'You see charities where it is about the people that founded them, and that can be tricky.'

Being valued is crucial. Ceinwen acknowledges that in some ways she is now in a privileged position. She doesn't need the flattery of being asked to 'give her views' for free, nor is she reliant on bits and pieces of money to have what she calls 'my brain sucked by the NHS'.

'I have got to the point where I know I have expertise to offer. The system does not yet respect patient leaders as people who should be employed or paid to do this work well; it doesn't happen. At most, people get an honorarium per day and are not treated as paid consultants as part of an ongoing programme.'

'We are modelling a different sort of service provision – setting up the market stall outside the citadel.' You bang your head against fewer walls out here.

It's also notable that they are working with young people and online. Social media has been important (though she admits that they have needed to move beyond Facebook towards newer digital platforms). 'We haven't cracked it yet.' But you feel she will.

DEALING WITH POWER

Dominic Makuvachuma Walker

'If you feel you are a freak and a force of nature, want to explore that potential, pulse and aliveness, let's have a conversation... Life gives you lemons; you make lemonade.'

In 1994, Dominic, who stands at only 5 feet 7 inches, was working as the 'doorman' at a 'blues' party for reggae lovers (who were mainly black people) in London, which he describes as a 'shebeen': 'You know the size of me! I had the people skills, made it easy for people to pay and get in. It was around the time of the Stephen Lawrence murder; it was not unusual to have parties in like-minded people's homes. You donated £2–3, booze was sold in cans.' His voice quietens as he continues.

'There was a man a few floors above in the same block of flats who didn't like black people, didn't like the noise and he was trained in the Territorial Army. He put on a balaclava, picked up a machine gun and petrol can and decided he was going to stop the noise and kill us all.' What happened next has both haunted Dominic and made him the man he is now.

'A white man decides he doesn't like the music, so he decides he's going to kill us all? Fucking hell.'

The assailant walked in, did a recce of the building, went back to his flat, dressed up and clutched a machine gun (that turned out to be a replica) and a firebomb (which was very real).

When he returned to the party, he cleared out the passage in order to throw the petrol bomb. Dominic was the closest person to him, pressed up against a wall. 'The guy saw me frozen there and put down his tank, lit it up, dropped it and kicked it into the house to accelerate the fire. Right in my face.'

Worse, Dominic saw a young mother jump out of a window to her death. The firebombing became a murder investigation. Dominic became the first witness for the prosecution.

He suffered third-degree burns to his arms and superficial burns to his face. And, unsurprisingly, PTSD. 'I was at the window when she dropped, but my mind does not allow me to see that. In that same way, I cannot record some of what I did and needed to do in order to survive after that.'

At the time of the firebombing, Dominic was a 27-year-old Zimbabwean actor who had come over to Guildford to film *The Power of One* and then stayed on to try and make it in the London film industry. He was at first impressed with the racial tolerance he witnessed in London, although he later witnessed the rise of racial tensions in the mid-1990s.

'I was on an adventure. I saw a different kind of white people to the Rhodesian racists I'd been used to, who contributed to a life of knowing my place. It was a fascinating shock to walk down Oxford Street and for nobody to give a shit about me being black. But it was a funny time, Stephen Lawrence had just been killed. I didn't realise I would become so mixed up in that world.'

The police took a keen interest in Dominic's case as part of the murder investigation. But the investigation focused on the murder as an individual response of someone triggered by the noise of the party, stripped of its racial context: 'The court system and press coverage seemed to be colluding with the racism by making it invisible. So, you can imagine the impact and additional forces in my head. This was more than just physical burns and hurt. My struggles during this time were now also psychological. They seemed to be saying: "We know the guy had Nazi paraphernalia, was in Combat 18 [a neo-Nazi terrorist organisation] and a known racist, but we are not going to look at that, because that's going to prejudice the client. So, let's just focus on the fact that he was annoyed by the noise."'

'And I am saying, "You fuckers, he's a racist." The activist in me was activated. You don't wake up at 2am and put on a balaclava and hold a machine gun and petrol bomb because you've been woken up by the fucking noise.'

Dominic lived with the mixed emotions of paranoia, rage and PTSD for several years. 'I wanted justice. I did not know how to channel the anger.' They did catch the assailant within 48 hours of the incident, but, given the way his mind was racing, Dominic couldn't be sure they had got the right man. He suffered flashbacks and hyper-vigilance: 'When I saw a white man I saw the same eyes. How do I know they got the right guy? He had a balaclava. No one saw his face. It was not a nice place. My narratives were odd; I was volatile to the point of endangering other people.'

He goes on: 'But there is always a context. Always an antecedent. If society created a monster called Dominic, I think that's a story that needs to be told. Don't talk to me about having a chip on my shoulder when you don't know what happened. You need to understand the lemons we get dealt. It takes time for it to become lemonade.'

His burns took a long time to heal and needed plastic wrapping and creams. He could not use his hands, could not work and could not claim benefits for a long time because his assumed name was not traceable to his National Insurance contributions from his working life between 1991 and 1994. Meanwhile, his rage simmered: 'I wanted revenge. I remember having strong urges to plan and execute the bombing of the local magistrate court. That's what made me realise I was fucked up in my head.'

Dominic recalls his early years of looking for all kinds of jobs to survive in London. For example, he worked as a cleaner in a Turkish restaurant for £100 a week, half of which funded him to attend a summer drama school and the other half went on rent and a travel card, with £1.20 a week left over.

'My National Insurance contributions up to this period were finally linked with my assumed name after an interview with the Department of Social Security, and this was the first stages of legitimising Dominic Walker (not Dominic

Makuvachuma). I was attending the day centre during this time and unable to work because I was a mess – physically and emotionally.'

'In 1997 I was arrested for attempting to obtain a British passport with false information – that spelt the beginning of the slow death of Dominic "Walker", who I had created to serve the purpose of anonymity. I was imprisoned for 18 months (reduced to nine months on appeal) and came out in May 1998.'

He laughs: 'I think my tactics were genius, but I am not proud of it any more. Better to frame it like this: if survival is the name of the game, I would probably get high marks for it. If morality were to be the compass, I would fail dismally. I now measure myself by the latter.'

His son had been born while he was in prison and he had a new life to return to.

Reflecting on what he had done wrong, he is keen to stress both responsibility and the context: 'I had become this monster that I did not recognise, that did not know right from wrong, but I also had an acute sense of social injustice in this country and felt my mission and my core was good.' He continues: 'Don't judge someone with a criminal record. You must understand the story. I was not born that way.'

Dominic began attending a day centre for black people, where he got support and gradually rebuilt his shattered confidence. He appreciated the help he was getting and started to notice what was going on around him again. But he was still 'quiet as a church mouse – I just went in and out'.

And then one day he found his voice – both literally and metaphorically. There were proposals to move the centre to a purpose-built, improved location. But some attendees started spreading rumours of mismanagement. 'I knew what was happening from apartheid, the internalising of oppression. That had made me feel that I know my place, that I shouldn't take a piss, 'cos all toilets are for whites only. I saw that belief in inferiority manifesting in a different way.'

'I'm thinking, "Black people, shut up." We've got a new centre, let's celebrate. That's the first time I spoke, and somebody heard me. "Did you hear what he said?" I was coming out of my shell. And they started to encourage that.'

As Dominic resurrected his career, he began to find opportunities for his voice. He was invited to local events and asked to share his views on what the centre was doing as part of a transcultural project. This provided that all-important sense of purpose – not only was he expressing gratitude for what the centre had done, he also argued as to why it needed to remain a black-only service, drawing deeply on his own experiences: 'You look at what I went through. It does not become more vivid than that. When someone is trying to work through flashbacks, seeing a white man walking down the street and being hyper-vigilant, always thinking, "How do I know they've got the right guy?" You know we need safety.'

He started speaking more widely about equalities and race relations: 'That racial dimension of my case was quite explicit. And remains so. And I think it is hard-hitting even when I say it now. It's undeniable. That there is that hostility in race relations in our country. It just doesn't get that explicit usually. It simmers. I feel it, I know it is there.'

Sharing platforms with other speakers and meeting

others doing similar work locally bolstered his sense of purpose and connections to the community. In 1997, he met someone who helped him make his next 'quantum leap' – a trainer called Peter Fern. 'This guy said, "So, tell me about you." I wasn't used to people being interested in me. I told him I used to be an actor and his eyes lit up. And then I told him about the firebombing and prison life.'

Peter and Dominic created training and development programmes on race and culture with case scenarios for social care staff. Dominic drew on his background as a performing artist to create personas for the scenarios based on characters he had met interwoven with his own experiences. Crucially, these showed how mental health problems are caused by circumstances beyond one's control.

Things were coming together, and he was helping transform services and challenging the status quo – the actor and the activist had been resurrected. And he felt he was no longer watching his back; the hyper-vigilant state was receding: 'I was starting to get my life straight.'

Having met Simon Barnett, of Mad Pride, he was ushered onto a national stage. 'Simon was a white copper, real East End guy, used to be married to a black sister. He had the temerity to walk into a black day centre and I thought, "Who is this guy?" I felt infringed because of my shit, but he saw beyond colour.'

He told Dominic to up his game and took him into work-supporting organisations to set standards: 'And I was like, "Woah, this is a new world."' He learnt about mental health survivor organisations, health and social care systems and processes that he later used to his advantage in national work. He met other people who would become his gurus and mentors, such as Pauline Abbott-Butler, who had created the first Afro-Caribbean User-Survivor Forum, and its chair, Patricia Chambers, as well as Peter Beresford and David Creasey, all of whom were pioneers of the mental health service user rights movement.

Impressed by his passion and energy, I ask him midway through our discussion how he looks after himself. He laughs. 'If you want advice on how to look after yourself in all this, I am not the person to come to. If you feel you are a freak and a force of nature, want to explore that potential, pulse and aliveness, let's have a conversation about how to manage that. But you can burn out quickly. It's about finding that balance.'

We return to his career. In 2003, he was confident enough of his potential to make that difficult leap from benefits to employed work. 'I was aware of a certain learned help-lessness kicking in.' His first break was to join the Social Perspectives Network (a coalition of service users/survivors, carers, policy makers, academics, students and practition-ers interested in how social factors contribute to people becoming distressed, and in promoting people's recovery) as a part-time manager, and then he joined the Afiya Trust (a national charity that works to reduce inequalities in health and social care provision for people from Black and Minor-ity Ethnic (BME) communities). During this time, he also managed to get a BSc in health service management and then went to a large national charity, Together, to work on community development and wellbeing.

By now, he could feel momentum in his career. 'I thought,

"Life gives you lemons; you make lemonade." That's the logic.' And for the first time in a long time, he felt a sense of gratitude that still comes over when he talks: 'I was using my skills, earning a living, able to influence. That did not sound like an unfair exchange.'

He joined the national charity Mind in 2012. He felt that this large mental health charity was losing its way and was not doing anything for black people. They were looking for someone with 'lived experience', and over the last five years he has pioneered work on peer support and on how local groups could influence health services. This was at a time of huge changes to the way the NHS structured its commissioning functions, with PCTs being replaced by CCGs (smaller, ostensibly GP-led, local funding organisations).

Dominic's belief in the ability of local people – leaders – with lived experience to lead the way was pivotal. Mind, together with the National Survivor User Network (NSUN), looked at what was going on with peer support all over the country. They linked with local Mind groups and went digital – creating first a Facebook page with 5000 people as peer supporters and then developing an independent organisation that migrated to more sophisticated online platforms. His work revolved around a small, flexible team that included researchers who had lived experience.

It was an exciting time: 'We were dumped into things. We didn't have a flat-pack of what we would do; it emerged. People came along for the ride. It was giddy but fun.'

Out of the scoping-best-practice work, they created Peer-Fest, a now annual celebration of peer support, replete with 'music, prosecco, choirs... Who said this work had to be dull?'

And the important factor? 'I made sure we listened and took action. I take some cred for that. I am not good at knowing when I have made an impact. That's a confidence thing. But we created a bit of a critical mass and a reputation as "the guys that do and listen".'

Dominic remembers groups arguing about what the PeerFest logo should look like and whose organisational name should go where – a common experience for those in partnership work. 'Then someone rushed in and said, "Hey, stop that bloody bickering, the event is full." We didn't need a logo for the flyer.'

From these experiences, Dominic has grown into a confident leader – at least that is how he appears to others. He has developed solid conceptual frameworks for what he does. He describes how there were three circles to the Mind work: independent, peer-led groups doing peer support, local organisational-led peer support and then a wider circle of celebration and sharing of learning. 'Imagine those three circles converging – that's the liminal space where my team operates. It feels a bit shaky. We were custodians of that space, holding it, but letting innovation happen. Organisations are not ready to work in that space, but that is where innovation happens.'

On listening to this homegrown wisdom, one gets an inkling as to why patient or user leaders are so essential. You wonder whether the ability to hold the vision through uncertainty – indeed, seeing that simmering cauldron of potential as critical – is something that comes uniquely from lived and bitter experience.

'So here I was managing in health services – never my

first option. The calling was a series of things that happened in my life that left me thinking I need to understand how the system works in order to understand how they could get it so wrong where they did and how they could get it right or improve it. So, I'm here as a leader, not by choice, but by circumstance.'

He goes on: 'The hallmarks of what is now being called "patient leader" were there from the time I got firebombed. But, in fact, I used to do leadership; it came to me very early in my childhood – in my school, I did fundraising for charities and local community work. But before my experiences in this country, I was more commercial-sector oriented than doing what's right. My experiences have sharpened my desire to do the right thing and challenge what is not right – things that are unfair, discriminatory. I became an activist because of my lived experience.'

Unfortunately, physical health problems continue to plague his life. A few years ago, he had to have an operation to remove a tumour at the back of his chest and he now has diabetes and myasthenia gravis (involuntary eye movements).

He talks about patient leadership, a concept he was not initially comfortable with, having come from the mental health movement that sees the phrase 'patient' as redolent with meanings around passivity in relationship to professional power. 'It began to make sense in the way you [David Gilbert] were talking about.'

Like most other patient leaders, the motivation for the work stems from wanting to support improvement 'so that anything bad that happened to me should not happen to the next person. And anything that was good – exceptional – must be replicated across the country or across the globe. That's my goal.'

'Because you [David Gilbert] have given me that voice. Always. To keep it real. Not just for me but for others, for fairness and justice in the world.' And he is keen to move beyond national work: 'We don't live on a little British island. This should be a global platform. I witnessed my brother die of AIDS in Zimbabwe and could not do anything about it. Because I was an "overstayer" in the UK, I could not send medicines or bring him over. I watched him die at 39. I heard him speak, phoned him the day he died, his wife saying, "Dennis is not breathing." I need to connect to those global challenges and conversations.'

He has learned, intimately, of power and talks about finding the lever, the optimal place to shift the most with the least effort. 'We – patients, users and carers – have been spectators for a very long time. In fact, we still are. Professionals and institutions don't give us an opportunity to point out those levers we have seen because they are about totally rattling the status quo.'

I ask him whether he feels he has made a difference. There is the longest pause of our two-hour conversation: 'That's intertwined with my low self-esteem, I can't easily judge the impact I have. I know I do this work with integrity and sincerity. I can't stand back and see – someone must embrace me. But yes, I do enjoy it and feel a purpose and can feel some impact.'

He sees peer support as modelling the sort of change he wants to see, where you can give and receive. 'That changes the purpose of going to a service. Right there. At a stroke. There, my relationship with services is being challenged and changed. When I hear of the resistance to peer support, I know exactly what is being resisted, that power dynamic that is being shifted with peer support.'

Dominic weaves effortlessly between his personal experience, the work of people like himself and issues of power. He is sceptical of how national agencies appropriate social movements. He has seen it in peer support and wonders whether it might happen with patient leadership. 'We need to share our own insight; we have so much experience. If we were to find a way to tap into that knowledge, we could easily solve the problems of the NHS.'

'I believe we have to live with all our lemons and say, "Gosh, I've got lots of resources to make lemonade; it's not a problem." It becomes a problem because of how you look at it. How you look at me. I'm not a problem. I have to deal with it, and that's very resourceful by the way.'

He stresses that this capacity and capability should not be ignored a second time (as it often is when being a patient) as patient leaders enter the wider arena: 'We need to watch out for networks controlled by professionals. And we need also to keep an eye out for exclusion as a network grows. There is often a need to contain as things get bigger and that can lead to exclusion. I have some alarm bells ringing when I see NHS agencies taking over.'

Underlying these suspicions is a keen sense of what Dominic calls 'institutional arrogance', which he believes 'stops people listening'. For him, resistance lies in the way professionals are trained: 'I wouldn't be surprised to hear docs say, "I've spent years studying this, how can a patient teach me anything?" This is built in to health system design. You're trained to diagnose in such and such a way, bring scientific solutions to a problem, and so you play God in a certain way.'

He is generous about alliances with professionals and mentions 'transformational professional leaders who get it' as crucial allies. 'But I think we need to keep focused on the prize – the equity of status of the patient. I'm going to be done to? No more! That's gone. Forget co-design, we should all be together co-producing.'

'The work is energy sapping,' Dominic says. But he laughs: 'It's not surprising that when a mere pleb tells you that "your system is flawed, guv", it's a bit of a body blow isn't it?'

OUTSIDER-INSIDE

David Gilbert

Sure, I knew how to challenge people and wage battle on professionals. But could I help?

I am the youngest of three brothers. I wanted them to leave me alone. But I also wanted them to play with me, to love me. I wanted both freedom and belonging.

Therein lies the key to my career of activism – that and the catalysing effect of my hero worship of Billy Bremner, pugnacious captain of my Leeds Utd of the 70s, John McEnroe, magical and irreverent US tennis player, and Steve Biko, South African anti-apartheid activist.

This personal background also instilled, I think, the need to promote healing relationships and to foster support amongst wounded individuals. It is a contradictory set of values. Or, in ridiculous NHS leadership jargon that always coarsens language, 'there is a tension' between my values.

My values around independence fed my campaigning for change. I had also gone through a bad back injury that put me out of all sport apart from competitive swimming, my parents' divorce and my granny going senile when I was 15. At that time, I 'stayed together' and was not seemingly affected. I was a rock. Or so I liked to believe.

I joined Third World First and War on Want at university and wrote an essay on thalidomide (which moved me powerfully, as it affected my generation of 1962-born kids). I then wrote a dissertation on the evils of the pharmaceutical industry promoting anabolic steroids to malnourished children in developing countries. I had a burning sense of injustice – it's a younger brother thing (aka 'It's not fair, why do they get more roast potatoes, stay up late, go to the US...?').

In hindsight, it was also a rekindling of my mother's experiences as a kindertransport refugee from Nazi-occupied Vienna. And perhaps the wider Jewish experience of other ancestors. My great-aunts were communist Zionists. My great-great-great-grandfather, Rabbi Samson Raphael Hirsch, founded neo-orthodox Judaism in the face of assimilation and the reform movement in the late 19th century. My amazing uncle Robin supported the causes of outsiders all his life.

My first real opportunity to help make a difference came after meeting Charles Medawar – a one-man campaigning phenomenon who worked from a lock-up North London garage. He gave me my first job after uni, researching who had shares in the tobacco industry (the Labour Party, cancer charities, the Church of England, etc.). That was a blast, in more senses than one, for a heady young lad who spilled the beans on corporate hypocrisy. We made the front pages.

Charles then linked me up to Health Action International (HAI), a network of non-governmental organisations around the world lobbying for more openness and transparency in medicines licensing and better regulation of medicine safety and promotion. This modelled the incredible Infant Baby Food Action Network (IBFAN), which gave me my first taste of the power of networking and of consumer boycotts (against Nestlé) that helped change policy and practice and saved lives.

I met the amazing Andrew Chetley (who would be best man at my wedding) and with Ana Blanco-Chetley we wrote *Problem Drugs*, an information and education pack that brought together the evidence of safety and effectiveness of drugs that were widely sold in developing countries. It was translated into two dozen languages and went to three editions. Through it I met all sorts of amazing people all over the world who were activists for change and community leaders – patient groups and professional groups working together to shift the status quo. The precursors of the evidence-based medicine brigade – people who did stuff as well as wrote about it.

And then, at 22 years old, I became HAI's assistant coordinator in the Netherlands. I was at the gateway to a buzzing and budding international career. But then I began to blow it, bit by bit.

I now realise, after years of therapy, that I was ready for the fall. I had not in any way processed what had happened at age 15. As one healer I went to see put it, I was a 'skater on thin ice'. I was charming, bright and driven. But...

I'd started to have anxiety attacks while working with Charles. I remember him correcting my work and me struggling with stomach aches on waking. At uni, an essay on the Cold War (oh the irony!) had me taking seven tomes out of the library and then sitting in front of them crying, paralysed by the immensity of what I had to do, in a cold rented room in rainy Moss Side, Manchester. In my last year at uni, I found myself banging my head against the front door to rid myself of the pain of intrusive negative thoughts inside my head. The river of anxiety ran through me.

I was offered the HAI coordinator post, but turned it down, went back to London, mooched around and got a job in Neal's Yard Remedies in its early days. I was even offered a job in its small South London factory helping to make organic shampoos! I turned that down too. I got into all sorts of New Age activities. I was beginning to believe in angels and that chanting would cure cancer. I was also falling in and out of love with increasing regularity. Head banging on walls. Leaving others to do likewise, probably.

Then, I crashed and burned. I fell apart during what should have been a romantic rendezvous in San Francisco – an apt place for the earth to be rent asunder. I got an early flight home, leaving my then girlfriend perplexed.

The years between 1987 (the year of the great storm) and 1993 were... I am struggling to word it...

For six years, I was in a continual agonising mental state. My brain had short-circuited. I could not think beyond my own thinking. I was paralysed by a wiring so intense that it suffocated me. I would have a thought about, say, a flower. Then another part of my brain would say, 'You are thinking of a flower,' then another, 'You are thinking about thinking,' then another would criticise, 'You should not be thinking about thinking,' and then an exhausted part of the brain would say, 'I can't cope with this,' and, finally, 'Kill yourself.' These 'loops' occurred within a fraction of a second and then repeated immediately. I would tell everyone who would listen (and many who would not) about my loops and burned my friends out too. The pain went on and on. I can honestly say there was no let up. For six years, day in, day out. It was excruciating.

My friends and family could not cope. I went in and out of various therapeutic communities (none of which could cope either) and psychiatric institutions. And my experiences of the mental health system exacerbated my anger about injustice – I saw first hand what bad care looked like. Dismissive attitudes, bullying of patients, inadequate support, you name it.

Once, I was sitting in a psychiatric ward with nothing to do – the lunch had been awful, the occupational therapist had been sacked (so no activities that afternoon) and the ward seemed full of screaming folk. A doctor strolled onto our bay and gave a perfunctory nod before gingerly pulling on the curtain rail beside my bed. Even in my disturbed state, I could see his behaviour was odder than mine. I asked him what he was doing. 'Just checking to see if you could do anything stupid,' he replied, before walking back down the corridor. I was left contemplating the sudden and unintended addition to my range of 'treatment' options.

Meanwhile, three fellow in-patient friends of mine died. Lesley-Anne had choked to death on her food while unsupervised after she had left the psychiatric unit and gone to a nursing home (she had earlier been paralysed from the neck down through a failed suicide attempt). Steve had gone to his caravan and hanged himself. And Larry had drowned himself in the local reservoir.

I have drawn on these experiences throughout my subsequent career. For me, when I read later that in-patient suicide prevention targets included 'removing all non-collapsible curtain rails', I remembered that doctor who had checked my curtain rail. And my friends who had died.

All those deaths had occurred away from the in-patient environment, so the unit would have passed its inspection by having removed ligature points. It might also have been congratulated on its risk policies. This was 'hitting the target and missing the point'. The unit had responded to the caravan and reservoir deaths by locking the doors at 8pm. This deprived me of my one visitor, a local chaplain, who I could only get to see at 9pm. Nights became a pressure cooker of aggravated emotions – the consequence of this lack of trust and forced containment felt unsafe. I wonder whether dialogue between us in-patients and staff about what makes for a safe environment might have saved my friends.

Designing services without involving service users is a waste of time – worse, it is unsafe in the broadest sense. I am still angry.

However, poor experiences are not only for storytelling. Nor are they only to be used as admonishment – that way lies initial necessary change and power shifts, but risks long-term polarisation and maintenance of the us-and-them mentality, which I believe should be overcome.

During those interminable years, I learned more about what matters to all of us who have been through life-changing illness, injury or disability – things like quality of life, respect and dignity, access, continuity, support for carers, care beyond meds, ability to get back on your own two feet, how to look after yourself. These things matter whether you have diabetes or schizophrenia, cancer or depression.

Furthermore: you do not know until you have lived it what truly matters. In the crucible, you also learn about what it means to be truly stripped of humanity, your identity, your hopes, your relationships. These sorts of sensations, feelings, emotions – call them what you will – are the invisible threads that connect all patient leaders together, in my opinion. And are why we need to be part of every single decision that is made in the health service. Who else has skin in the game?

I also saw great care. One day, Dr Ikkos, my consultant psychiatrist, said, 'I hear you used to do work in the field of pharmaceutical policy and were a community development activist in developing countries. I see you are a good writer and used to teach doctors about the side effects of drugs. Maybe you can help me.' He got what mattered.

I walked into Napsbury Hospital with Dr Ikkos to deliver a talk to his medical students on pharmaceutical policy and the benefits and risks of psychotropic medicines (the evidence and my experience). I walked into the place I imagined I would end up a long-term inmate and where I thought I would die.

I got up in front of an audience of future doctors and they listened to what mattered to me: how the medicines I had taken had ballooned me in size so that I was even more bereft of confidence; how the environment on the ward was making me feel more unsafe; how I had lost my identity because I was unable to do what mattered most – write and campaign on health issues.

I realised then that 'care and treatment' is about a professional thinking more about life and less about what the 'service' can offer. I walked into that vast Victorian asylum as a patient and walked out a professional and a human. Because one doctor had dared to ask 'What matters?' and, more importantly, had listened. And, even more importantly, had done something about it.

I found new friends and wonderful staff. Dorothea, the cook, kept my roast lamb warm after I had run away from the unit for a few hours. Mandy, the receptionist on the unit, often sat me down next to her at reception with a cup of tea if I was feeling particularly anxious. Once, she offered me tea, 'two sugars this time', after I'd witnessed a friend putting his fist through a window.

I remember once being allowed off the ward to go to the main hospital cafeteria. As I lined up for a cup of tea, I noticed a man holding hands with his small son. I recall distinctly the voice in my head: 'You will never be a father.' And then the deep sorrow that followed this punitive thought that I took to be truth.

And then, in June 1991, I met Susan. She was from Finland and had lost her two-year-old son, Nicholas, to a complex congenital heart defect. We first met over a cup of chamomile tea and bowl of cornflakes in the kitchen on the ward.

We clung together in the wreckage and provided solace for each other during long days over months. Often, we retreated into the laundry room, overlooking the hospital car park. It provided us with a place of sanctuary removed from the chaos and unpredictability of the ward environment. It was the only facility free of cigarette smoke and the TV's noise.

Many staff wondered how long such a relationship would last. A year later, we moved in together, a flat above a dry cleaners near a great fish-and-chip shop that we still go to. Best of all: we got married in 1997 and have two wonderful boys, Samuel and Adam, now 19 and 15.

Recovery may be an endless task. For many people with mental health problems, it is a contested term. For me, it was a miracle.

In the summer of 1993, I could do more, read more than a paragraph in a book without my intrusive thoughts making me despair quite so much, swim again for ten minutes before being driven out by my 'loops' and maintain a relationship with a woman I loved who was healing slowly too. I also began an MSc in Health Psychology, which gave me back some structural discipline.

I remember being in Finland with Susan by a lake that summer. I knew my mother and step-father were retiring from London and moving to Scotland. I would fill buckets with fresh water and carry them back to the cottage. I felt my thoughts slow down and a space opening up inside me. I returned to the UK to find my caring psychiatrist worrying about whether I was now about to shift into psychosis!

This was actually a dangerous time, looking back – another learning point that I have tried to use in my career: getting better or living with a health condition is not a linear process. And my experience of mental health recovery at one point found me 'doing better' (this being the yardstick for discharge from the service) but still feeling like crap most of the time.

I think this is the most important thing I have learned about mental health problems – that one's behaviour precedes feelings. In other words, I had to rebuild good habits. But the lure of the old symptoms, perhaps my neuro-physiological wiring (I am a fan of the Alexander Technique), pulled me back into feelings that were unreliable. The self-talk was still overwhelming, even when I was obviously able to better live in society.

Once, after a lecture on the MSc Health Psychology course – a module on the 'biological basis of behaviour' – I found myself sobbing in the toilet, perfectly understanding the intellectual basis for what was happening to me, and wanting to die. My self-talk was: 'OK, I can do more stuff, but if I am going to feel like this, then what is the point?'

My mind was tricking me into believing that my current state of cognition and feeling would be perennial. This itself caused me to relapse into what I felt was an even worse state. I would constantly say to people, 'I am back to square one.' And, of course, I was terrified of landing back in the psychiatric unit.

I had lost many friends along the way, those who had felt too unsafe around me, or felt they 'could not do anything' and could not bear to see me in the state I had been in. But one or two hung on. One or two had faith. Susan, of course. And people like Andrew and Ana.

I also know that my white, male, middle-class privilege allowed me back into society more easily than others.

It was beautifully ironic for this Jew to be supported by some true Christians. One was Robin Gold, who, when others had given up on me, continued to offer his flat as refuge from the psychiatric unit and often said, 'David, this too shall pass. You will be a great man.' I am not sure he was reliable in his judgement! But I wish he had lived long enough to read this book.

I also met Margaret Burrows. She had taken pity on me once when I had stumbled into a church service after wanting a break from the psychiatric unit. She says she saw me surrounded by kindly old women after the service, drinking coffee in the church hall. She felt she needed to rescue me! Over the next few months and years, we became friends and I got to know her family. Susan and I see her like a 'granny' to our children and we remain very close almost 30 years later.

Very gradually in late 1993, my thoughts and feelings became quieter and less incessantly punitive. This followed in the wake of my more intentional behavioural habits and the 'loops' gradually subsiding. I began the slow 'normalising' journey back to life. I had been six years in the system and I was a stranger to life.

And professionally, I was left up shit creek. Unlike many patient leaders, I had had a career in health activism before my illness. And, maybe because of that, I didn't have a choice but to go back into it, fuelled by what I had experienced first hand.

I had met Elsie Lyons and Jacqui Lynskey during my time in the psychiatric unit. They became friends and allies and were founding members of the 'Barnet User Group' (now called Barnet Voice for Mental Health) – see www.inclusionbarnet.org.uk/barnet-voice-for-mental-health). They were my inspiration for getting more involved and resurrecting my own professional confidence.

I volunteered at my local Mind mental health charity and became the chair. Then I became a member of the Community Health Council – the original 'statutory voice' for patients and the public. I helped the local health authority with its 'Care in the Community' developments and am still proud that we helped close Napsbury Hospital, an old Victorian asylum, and developed really good stuff for service users across the borough (although I sometimes wonder where much of the money went – land deals I expect).

My return to paid work came in 1994, when I borrowed a friend's ill-fitting suit (I was still fat from drugs) and bluffed my way through an interview for the Consumers in Europe Group, claiming that my six years 'away' had been as a freelance consultant (boy, had I been freelance!). For six months, I somehow blagged my way through work on consumer rights and EU food policy.

My big break then came when I went to the Consumers' Association (publishers of *Which?*) as their lead on medicines and complementary therapies. My confidence was coming back, but I still was not open about my mental health experiences, except with close colleagues. And my skills developed – as a clearer and cleaner writer, as a more scrupulous researcher and as a medicines policy expert. But

I was still an angry campaigner and outsider. Sure, I knew how to challenge people and wage battle on professionals.

But could I help?

At the King's Fund, a health policy think-tank, I learned more about evidence-based practice, providing better information for patients, qualitative analysis and, crucially, that not all health professionals are the enemy. I met mavericks who were good to me – particularly the late, great and incredibly kind service user advocate Bob Sang and my life-long friend Mark Duman.

I came to realise that I was decent at bringing 'both sides' together – that I was a natural connector, what one person later described as an 'animateur' (I had to look that word up).

I am also a writer and poet, thus I was beginning to bring different parts of my broken self back together: critic–survivor–connector–creator... Those of us who have been affected by life-changing stuff may recover or rebuild – for me, the better word is 'reintegrate' or 'reconnect' – and thus serve as a personal microcosm of the healing needed around us.

My eclectic – some would say 'mongrel-like' – career unfolded. I moved from the King's Fund to a consultancy organisation, the Office for Public Management (OPM), where I learned how to perform under pressure. My role was as 'stakeholder engagement' fellow. Posh title, tough job. We were to support NHS organisations to 'engage' with the people who used their services, communities and citizens. Back then, in the late 1990s, there was money sloshing around the NHS. And we did great work. I remember running a Citizens' Jury in Leicester around the contested closure of an A&E department. There were 120,000 people who had signed a 'hands-off-our-hospital' petition – and two high-profile MPs on 'opposite sides', both battling to save 'their' hospital.

After we did our work, the local newspaper headlined with 'Both Sides Win'. We had found a way through proper engagement to come up with proposals that unlocked a deal. We were knocked off the front page that week only by 'Barn Owl Falls Down Sewer', which did upset me.

At OPM, we had targets called 'billable' days. We had to, if I remember rightly, bring in 13.5 days' worth of daily fees per month and worked with amazing colleagues who taught me the craft of organisational development, change management, true facilitation and evaluation. I loved it, particularly my little team of bright-eyed believers in co-production, led by the wonderful Kai Rudat (who died far too young).

In 2001, we developed 'Signposts' for the then National Assembly for Wales (see www.wales.nhs.uk/publications/signposts-e.pdf) – one of the first and, in my opinion, still one of the best resource guides for people undertaking patient and public engagement.

One of the OPM directors, Greg Parston, once brought me in and told me, 'You're charming, people like you, you're good at relationships. Now get smart, wear a suit and close the deals.' A perspective on where my strengths and weaknesses lay, and still lie. I still only have two suits; one is ripped at the ankle.

The best job I ever had (until now) came after OPM. The Bristol heart scandal (when babies died at high rates after cardiac surgery at the Bristol Royal Infirmary) led to the Kennedy Inquiry. This, in turn, led to the establishment of a slew of NHS quangos (back then people liked them) including the National Institute for Health and Care Excellence (NICE) (still going!), the National Patient Safety Agency and the Commission for Health Improvement (CHI) (in 2001), the first independent inspectorate for the NHS. I became CHI's 'head of patients and the public', overseeing a strategy called 'Nothing about us without us', which tried to ensure we focused on what mattered when we did inspections.

It was a bright, passionate, friendly organisation with the best set of directors I have ever seen. Led by Peter Homa, I was managed by the best boss I have ever had, Jocelyn Cornwell (others have come very close, but sorry...). This was partly because she gave me support to be my very best professionally – I had freedom to develop the role, yet clear and incisive support when I needed it.

I became more purposeful, I think. I certainly became more pragmatic. The work we did at CHI was trailblazing. One of the things that CHI did, amongst a whole heap of extraordinary stuff, was to put patient and public engagement as one of the core things that we inspected. These days it does not have the prominence in inspections and regulation that it did. And the way we supported organisations – the model for engagement we offered, as it were – I believe helped trusts to do it better. It was not punitive. And part of my role was to co-design and co-deliver training for general 'lay' and 'service user' inspectors. This was the foundation for the 'expert by experience' roles that the Care Quality Commission still uses.

During that time, I met Anthony Hewson, the deputy chair of CHI. He had a son with cerebral palsy. He once made the best speech I had ever heard about the blending of personal and professional expertise – very emotional and passionate. But he came off stage visibly exhausted. I asked him for advice on how to disclose my own story and use my expertise as an integral part of my role. He said that we have to 'use our stories judiciously' to make our strategic points. He also said that the emotional energy needed to make a speech like that is huge – the sense of vulnerability in public disclosure should not be underestimated. I have never forgotten those words.

I summoned up the strength then to tell Jocelyn about my mental health problems and decided I would more fully come out and 'own' the hard-won wisdom I had gained about mental health, illness and the care system. I decided that I needed to see those as an 'asset', not as a deficit. I was human and multifaceted, and the depth of my being that had been touched during my illness, my knowledge of what the mind was capable of in extremis, were to be my touchstone.

Jocelyn said two things that have stood the years when I told her about my mental health. First: 'It's not as important as you think it is. You are a human being and professional first and foremost.' She followed this swiftly by saying: 'But I know how important it is for you, and for you to tell me. It is part of you.'

For me, this dual recognition – of my being able to bring back to work my life skills and my professional skills that I had lost or that had been temporarily frozen, coupled with reframing my ill health experience as expertise – made all the difference.

This is what we bang on about. This is what we can't yet seem to get health professionals to acknowledge – we are *both*. Human and Patient. Human with our life and professional expertise. Thus equal. Patient, in the sense of having wisdom and insight forged in the caves of suffering. Our jewels are polished by our experience. I had six years of gruelling pain. It was equivalent to the best medical degree. Different. Equal. Full stop. That is when, at a deep level, I realised that patients can be, or are, leaders – actually years before we coined the term.

Looking back on it now, the rest is mere knowledge. Which anyone can get.

In 2003, I led work at CHI to gather the learning about patient and public engagement that we had learned as an inspectorate, before it changed to the Healthcare Commission. Our report was called 'I2I: Involvement to Improvement' (see www.wales.nhs.uk/sites3/Documents/420/Sharingthe LearningonPPIfromCHIswork.pdf) and showed that much of the involvement work done does not lead to impact – that there is a wall between many of the processes to learn from patients and doing something about it. This was my first major insight into the failings of the traditional approaches to empowering patients.

The following year, at the former NHSU (which was supposed to be a 'University for the NHS'), I met Jill Brunt, who had a background in adult education and learning and development. Our team was keen to develop a 'skills escalator' for patients at the same time as the concept of a 'skills escalator' was being developed for health professionals. We wanted to support opportunities for progression and learning for people who had had health conditions who wanted to get back into working to help change the system.

I developed this idea when at the former NHS Centre for Involvement, where I led a 'People Bank' of paid, trained and supported patients and carers to be 'consultant engagement advisors' to NHS organisations.

In 2008, I went on to develop my own consultancy, In-Health Associates, a small network of engagement specialists helping to support organisations to do effective patient and public engagement. I am so proud of the work I did, and still do, with InHealth Associates. I developed the Engagement Cycle on behalf of the wonderful Meredith Vivian at the Department of Health and while working with Croydon Primary Care Trust. The Cycle is used by commissioners to this day (see www.england.nhs.uk/improvement-hub/wp-content/uploads/sites/44/2018/06/The-Engagement-Cycle-Overview-PDF-final.pdf).

I learned more about healthcare policy and practice; about management structures and jargon; about how NHS policy can be wave after wave of reorganising the deckchairs and upholding leadership elites; about silo working and dismantling of professional humanism and, of course, about the failure of traditional engagement; about how we set up engagement to fail and preserve power. I have also been the victim of institutional bullying – how some organisations fail to practise what they preach. All the things we have talked about in this book.

And it is about humans doing great things – saving lives, doing their best, passionate and humane clinicians, an overwhelmingly amazing cadre of support staff – receptionists, administrators, porters, security staff, IT and HR departments, the lot. Lots right and lots wrong.

And then I started to meet people like me. People who had been through stuff, who knew stuff, who wanted to change stuff. For whom focus groups just would not do. They were brilliant, entrepreneurial, passionate, desiring purpose and wanting to connect their life and health wisdom. I was part of a group of misfits, mischievous mavericks on a pirate venture.

We met in cafes, the British Library Piazza and free office space where we could find it. And we shared our stories – like the Jewel Merchants around the camp fire.

I then met the extraordinary Mark Doughty in 2009 and we got on so well and had such complementary skills that we decided to work together. In 2010, Mark and I got our first opportunity to design and deliver a learning programme called the 'effective lay representative' programme for the NIHR CLAHRC Northwest London (National Institute for Health Research, Collaboration for Leadership in Applied Health Research and Care) – an unnecessarily long name for a necessary bunch of people! It is a partnership between Chelsea and Westminster Hospital NHS Foundation Trust and Imperial College London. Its main aim is to understand how evidence can be implemented to improve quality and outcomes in healthcare.

It was during these programmes that Mark and I honed our ideas and came up with the idea of patient leadership. It is hard to remember exactly, but I think what happened was we were running a session on the qualities needed to be an 'effective' lay representative. During the feedback, people called out words like 'vision', 'passion', 'integrity', 'resilience', 'humanity'... We realised then that these qualities were identical to 'leadership' qualities. I remember soon after phoning

Mark and us getting excited about the name 'patient leaders'. And very soon after that we came up with the idea for a Centre for Patient Leadership (CPL).

And a special mention for Rachel Matthews, Patient and Public Engagement and Involvement Theme Lead, who was alongside us every step of the way, helping to plan and deliver the CLAHRC work as we experimented and our ideas evolved. It was during these programmes that I met Patrick Ojeer and Alison Cameron.

Soon after that, Jeremy Taylor of National Voices sponsored a programme for some incredible 'patient-user leaders' within the voluntary sector (including Dominic Makuvachuma Walker and Trevor Fernandes). Jeremy remained a staunch supporter of patient leadership ideas.

Our third lucky break as CPL was running a large-scale patient leadership programme with FPM across the East of England, for the then strategic health authority. We wrote a practical guide on patient leadership as part of that work (see http://engagementcycle.org/wp-content/uploads/2013/03/ Bring-it-on-40-ways-to-support-Patient-Leadership-FINAL-V-APRIL-2013.pdf).

We set up the CPL formally in 2012. As far as I am aware, nobody was yet using our term 'patient leader' or 'patient leadership' – we wrote the first series of articles about patient leadership in the *Health Service Journal* between July 2012 and August 2013.

Over the next few years, the CPL provided learning and development for several hundred people. I learned loads from Mark. His excellent personal learning and development work with professionals and patients continues under the auspices of the King's Fund.

But I got frustrated with the difficulty of building a business and with finding institutional buy in to the deeper ideas of systemic change – how we can create the opportunities for networks of patient leaders at local and national level. And, more frustratingly, I sensed that ideas were being plagiarised and co-opted.

I still have a vision of a national network of patient leaders, which was hatched over 15 years ago during the development of the 'skills escalator' at NHSU, the People Bank at the NHS Centre for Involvement, and during my time working with Mark at the CPL: I would like to see an independent, patient/carer-led network that offers opportunities, belonging and support for people like us – those of us who have life-changing illness, injury or disability.

Not just for those who want to work in the NHS to help improvement, but for emergent entrepreneurs like Michael Seres or David Festenstein, those who want to develop community projects or peer support, like Ceinwen Giles, and of course for campaigners and activists, like Alison Cameron. I want it to be a true community of like-minded patient leaders who could develop in the way they want to – in the direction of their dreams, fully supported by their peers.

Recently, we had the opportunity – NHS Improvement gave £120,000 to develop a patient leader network. A few of us tried to help. I volunteered the name 'The Snow Community', which stuck (after Rosamund Snow – see the introduction). Sadly, I felt I had to leave due to what I sensed were poor project management arrangements. Others did so too. I hear the idea of a national patient leader network rumbles on. Good luck to it. But for the moment my heart is elsewhere.

From my experience of working at national level, it seems hard for large institutions to avoid over-controlling and stifling such initiatives. For the time being, I am more invested in local work. When I look back at my career – apart from at CHI – local is where it's been at.

Then, five years ago, I got a call from Steve Laitner. Steve is a GP and a passionate believer in the patient leadership work. He previously commissioned CPL to run a series of patient leadership training programmes in the East of England. Now, he was advising four organisations in Sussex to form a partnership that would oversee and run services for people with MSK conditions.

Those partners were bidding to get £50m a year for five years from three CCGs: Brighton and Hove CCG, Mid-Sussex and Horsham CCG and Crawley CCG.

During the partnership discussions, they made a commitment to ensure that 'patients were at the centre', that 'people who use services should be in control of their own care and choices' and that 'shared decision-making' and 'self-management' should be cornerstones of the treatment offer within the local MSK clinics they wanted to set up.

Steve told me that, during the discussions, they were talking about how to do this properly, to go beyond the 'tick-box' engagement and traditional ways of doing things. They had been talking about how trusts usually have someone overseeing complaints in one department, someone working on patient engagement in another, someone setting up self-management programmes in another, and so on.

This is a mirror of how services fragment people's journey through the system. And all these sorts of roles are lowly paid and without much status. Furthermore, they usually report into different directorates and each may be only a small part of any one director's portfolio.

They were beginning to draw one of those 'organograms' – the beloved NHS diagram of structures with lots of dotted lines that try to prove how everything links up. Then, Steve said, 'Well, if you want to do things differently, and you really want to be patient-centred...how about doing this...?'

Then he drew a box alongside the two boxes that contained the words 'Clinical Director' and 'Managing Director' and wrote 'Patient Director'. Steve, although Jew(ish) always spoke about the Holy Trinity of leadership – Clinical, Managerial, Patient. Different. Equal. Shared decision-making manifested at executive level. And what became known as the Sussex Model of Patient and Carer Partnership was born.

Huge credit must go to those around the table – those from Brighton Integrated Care Services (BICs, now called HERE), Sussex Partnership NHS Foundation Trust, Sussex Community NHS Foundation Trust and Horder Healthcare. And the CCGs. They all agreed to go for it.

They also created another important role – that of 'self-management lead', who would come to lead support and development for wellbeing, self-management and shared decision-making. This role was filled by my close colleague and now friend, Chloe Stewart, who has been trailblazing along with others.

The partnership also spotted the need for a 'Patient and Carer Forum' alongside the other key 'governance committees' (e.g. Finance and Performance, Clinical Quality, Operations) to really make sure 'patient-centred' work was happening and to be a place for true dialogue at corporate level. And then they won the contract.

My role is to help the partnership focus on what matters. This includes embedding patient-centred cultures, systems and processes such that they become 'hardwired' and making sure we learn from, and act on, what patients think about services. It should not be forgotten that the partnership not only had to deliver services for hundreds of thousands of people, it also had to transform the way previous fragmented services had worked. As one colleague said at the time, 'It was like changing the engine in the plane while it was still flying.'

At the same time, given my disenchantment with traditional engagement, I want to support patients to enable them to be influential and valued partners in decision-making. Being a patient director has enabled me to experiment with a different approach to engagement.

From the establishment of our service, I have had an annual budget of £25,000 and we have trained and supported a core group of Patient and Carer Partners (PCPs) paid £150 a day, to be involved in improvement and staff training (e.g. leading workshops during staff conferences) and to be members of our regular Patient and Carer Forums alongside staff.

They bring professional and personal wisdom alongside their experiences of using our services. PCPs are not representatives or there to provide feedback but are 'critical friends' who check assumptions, ask questions, provide insights into reframing issues or identifying problems, change dynamics and model collaborative leadership.

My role is to broker opportunities in improvement or governance and support them to ensure they have the capacity and capability to be effective. PCPs augment other involvement and feedback work. This work has been developed during a period of intense operational pressures. During the past four years, the partnership has transformed the way MSK services are delivered and PCPs have been alongside as we have done so.

The first challenge in bringing people in was to be clear that they were more than storytellers and were there to do more than feed back on their experiences (we had other data for that) and that they should stay in the room – proving themselves well able to reframe problems, generate new solutions, model collaborative leadership and shift dynamics.

PCPs have been involved in several major improvement programmes: pain services redesign, fibromyalgia pathways, plans for shared decision-making, administrative systems, support for receptionists and call handlers and integration of physical and mental health provisions. More recently, they have led on their own projects, such as an 'accessible communication and information project', and we have just recruited four more PCPs. I hope that they will work with staff to introduce peer support for people with MSK conditions, and turn our clinic waiting rooms into 'information hubs'.

An early experience helped us to demonstrate benefits.

We were discussing how to communicate with patients about booking appointments. We were receiving lots of calls to cancel or change inconvenient appointments that we had booked for people.

A woman who had been through our service told us that our team phoned at inconvenient times to book appointments. She suggested that, instead, we send opt-in appointment letters and put her in the driving seat. Let her phone back when she had her diary in front of her and she could plan out her week. We experimented with the idea and it was successful, with patients and call handlers alike delighted with how it worked. If this approach were rolled out, we would save an estimated 3500 cancelled appointments per year.

Last year, PCPs were integral to one of our Commissioning for Quality and Innovation projects (CQUINs come with money from commissioners attached). They helped support administrative staff (call handlers and receptionists) to enhance patients' experiences, for example triggering improvements in waiting-room environments, changing role descriptions for receptionists so as to focus on patient-facing duties, and helping to design call-handling training.

That project has bloomed into one where support staff and patients are working together to improve how we gather information about the communication needs of patients, improve information provision and make clinics more accessible.

Slowly, PCPs have become trusted equals. It has not been easy and is dependent on clarity of role, shared understanding of purpose, demonstrating benefits and the perennial time, money, space, trust... All things the NHS has precious little of.

We have now made the next step – for PCPs to move from an improvement role into a more steady-state governance role. We are experimenting with PCPs on our multidisciplinary teams (MDTs). We want to model reflective dialogue that focuses on what patients and staff think matter and issues of quality and patient experience. We will evaluate the work and see whether it could be a model for other pathways.

As one clinician noted: 'This patient and carer partner work does improve relationships, but more importantly for me it simplifies processes, bringing everything back to our main purpose of care. We can easily become wrapped up in our medical mind and "fix-it" mentality without much reference or consideration to our actions, all with extremely good intentions.'

The role of patient director is still novel, and this particular model of patient partnership is an experiment. It has taken a long time to build relationships, do the ground work and make the case for a different model of engagement. We see now, and I know for sure, that patient leadership is both desirable and feasible in the NHS. It cannot be ignored any more. The future depends on political will.

One member of a MDT noted: 'It is possible to have a more person-centred healthcare service if people are open to working differently and widening their horizons as to where solutions to improvements may be. Patient partners hold an experience of the systems that we want to improve. We need commitment and adequate time allocated to exploring this from both sides to ensure that roots can grow and that they become part of the make-up of the healthcare service as much as any clinician or admin team member.'

During this time, it seems that my own sense of professional confidence has grown. I still try to challenge people and question assumptions, but I like to think that I have helped to create a safer environment in which to do so, within the office and with colleagues. I have grown to love being a patient director, and am proud that I have stuck to my guns – which is, of course, not the best analogy!

There are still challenges: we need to communicate better the work of the PCPs so people know what they can do (and, sometimes, what they can't do, because they don't have the support that staff take for granted); we need to make sure we close the loop on data – to monitor actions and impact; we need to make sure that patient engagement is built in at the beginning of all corporate improvement projects. And, for PCPs, we need to put in better learning and support so that they can be even more effective.

In the current frenzy surrounding NHS policy and practice, it is worth remembering that long-term improvements take time, space and trust. There are no quick fixes. Our work in Sussex demonstrates one novel approach to the challenges of rethinking engagement. It is predicated on the four steps that are necessary to renew engagement: to value what people bring; to establish different mechanisms for dialogue; to develop people's capabilities; and to provide new opportunities for the new breed of patient (or carer) leaders.

As time has gone on, we have come to articulate a Sussex

Model of Patient and Carer Partnership. I envisage it as a triangle – between the role of patient director (at executive level), Patient and Carer Forum (at corporate governance level) and PCPs (involved in improvement and governance). It is backed up by systems and processes to ensure the work becomes part of everyday practice.

We are eager to share learning. Our local work is beginning to change things big time. And the group of ten PCPs could become the nucleus of a wider network or community of practice.

The idea of patient directors in healthcare is also gradually spreading. As well as my counterpart, Anne Sabine, in the Sussex MSK Partnership (East), the inspirational Chief Executive of Sussex Partnership NHS Foundation Trust, Samantha Allen, has created posts for two 'User and Carer Leaders'. Deb Owen and Louise Patmore operate at senior level in its forensics team and on quality throughout the Trust respectively. And the first patient director beyond Sussex, Cristina Serao, is now to be found at the Camden MSK Service under the auspices of UCLH (the University College London Hospitals NHS Foundation Trust).

All of us are taking on the role in slightly different ways. But all of us are dedicated to the steadfast principle of making sure patients, service users and carers are equal partners in senior decision-making and creating opportunities for others in the design and delivery of services. We are available for a chat and in order to share learning!

Personally, I have not always found the role of patient director easy – my travails are well documented on my blog. I have had bouts of mental health problems (redolent of my horrid years) and have sometimes struggled to feel my own worth in this role. But it is blossoming into one of the most worthwhile professional experiences of my life.

Meanwhile, I have met dozens of other eager patient leaders via Twitter, and during my travels around the country, to Canada and more recently to Australia. The potential for a worldwide movement is strong.

I was introduced to my own favourite coalition for change in this arena by Carolyn Canfield, a tireless, compassionate and hugely intelligent voice for patients and carers. The Patient Advisory Network (see www.patientadvisors.ca) dub themselves 'patient and family advisors who use our experiences to help improve Canadian healthcare for all of us'. Its website, built on voluntary passion, provides resources, opportunities and discussion forums. It is a hive of shared buzzy wisdom. We could learn a thing or two from them.

Back home, at 57, the writing of a book has also allowed me some much-needed reflective space. I have spent more than half a lifetime in patient and public engagement. I still pinch myself that I survived, let alone thrived. I feel privileged to have come so far, and that I may have helped change things a bit. But I am tired, particularly of pushing things at national level.

I have started to drift back towards mental health work. I feel I owe it to myself and others to give more there.

I am an Associate of the incredible Centre for Mental Health (see www.centreformentalhealth.org.uk) and have started to work with Re:Create Psychiatry (see https://recreatepsychiatry.com), a user-led initiative that wants mental health services to be made more healing, more human and more creative for everyone. This builds on my passion for bringing users and professionals together through better conversations and creative dialogue.

But my favourite role of all is as Writer in Residence at the extraordinary Bethlem Gallery (see http://bethlemgallery.com). Situated on the grounds of the Bethlem Royal Hospital, the gallery provides a professional space for high-quality artwork and fosters a supportive artist-focused environment. I have never been in a place that so values people – as artists and human beings primarily – with mental health conditions. It is a beautiful space. I go there once a month and do very little except breathe in the energy, chat to artists and visitors, and write.

In fact, sometimes I think I would prefer to sit and write poetry all day. Maybe under a tree. My favourite childhood book was *Ferdinand the Bull.* I am beginning to graft a creative life onto my healthcare career and have started to run creative writing workshops and poetic collaborations (see https://futurepatientblog.com/2018/10/29/rewrite-creative-approaches-to-engagement).

At the same time, my own professional confidence is stronger than it has ever been. And that is only because my life and mental health expertise is coupled closely with my professional expertise. I can help integrate services, I think, largely because I mirror that very integration within me. This may be dreamy. But it feels true. And more true every day when I see those around me doing likewise. The gang is doing amazing things. And so are thousands of other 'patient leaders'. Often invisible, readily marginalised and frustrated. Everyday heroes.

Meanwhile, in my corporate role, in the last six months I have felt better able to support my amazing colleagues, strategically and operationally. I have been less adolescent and needlessly challenging when stressed. I like to think I am a tad more creative, solution focused and insightful. Less of a younger brother. I enjoy the work more and look forward to going into the office. What more could a boy – sometimes a man – want?

Looking back, I now wonder what might have happened if a patient director had been around when I was on the psychiatric unit. Might my three friends, Lesley-Anne, Steve and Larry, still be alive?

What if the jewels of wisdom and insight people bring back from the caves of suffering were truly and universally valued? How many others would be able to live and live well?

For now, we are still on the winding road towards the crumbling citadels. We can and will help heal the healthcare system.

I hope this book helps people along the journey.

You Didn't Tell Me

You didn't tell me there would be days when I could walk out
on a garden by a low stone wall and breeze from the Baltic.

You didn't tell me there would be chaffinches in the oak
and gentle hill curving down to the reeds, lake and an empty boat.

You didn't tell me there would be oars, that I could steer to middle water
overlooked by black and white storks in towering nests.

You didn't tell me there would be time to pull in the oars,
let drift and swirl, that distant bells could sound like glockenspiels.

You didn't tell me that shivery and jagged reflections of white trees
could settle themselves into distinct silver parallel lines.

You didn't tell me that I could return at any time to the jetty,
or that when I stood, a turquoise dragonfly could land on my arm.

David Gilbert

THE CONTRIBUTORS

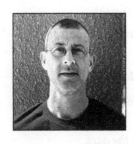 **Michael Seres** is the founder of 11 Health (www.11health.com), the world's first smart care platform focused on patients with long-term chronic conditions who are connected to medical bags. He was diagnosed aged 12 with the incurable bowel condition Crohn's disease. In late 2011 he became the 11th person to undergo a small bowel transplant in the UK at the Churchill Hospital in Oxford. More recently he is a two-time cancer survivor.

Michael started blogging about his journey and is a published author and patient mentor. He was the co-Chair of the NHS Digital Services User Council and helped implement the first Skype clinics in the UK. In 2015 he was announced as Stanford Medicine X's first Patient-in-Residence and is an Executive Board member. He is on the HIMMS UK Advisory Panel and is part of the US Health & Human Services advisory board on data accessibility.

Michael's Twitter handle is @mjseres.

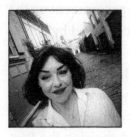

Kate James was originally born in the North East and is now most definitely a Hertfordshire girl. She has recently stunned herself by reaching 40 having never expected to make it. From a young age, Kate has learned to live with chronic ill health with severe complications but has been able to use her experiences of the health system to forge a career in the charity sector, bringing people together to make things better.

Kate is a true Jewel Merchant. She existed in the caves for a very long time but since connecting on a deep level with others who are also willing to share their jewels, she has found her wings and continues to work tirelessly to bring about positive chance.

Kate is honoured, if somewhat astonished, to be amongst the community that this book so eloquently illustrates and looks forward to being able to introduce her new nephew to her revolutionary family.

Kate's Twitter handle is @kookyK8.

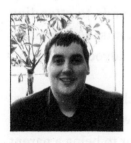

Dominic Stenning, who experienced drug and mental health challenges from a young age, has been involved with his local trust, Cambridgeshire and Peterborough Foundation Trust (CPFT), as a patient leader and expert by experience. He is also a member of the East of England Citizens' Senate, which was one of the first of its kind to be established. He was on the steering group of nine experts by experience, working on the Barker

Commission, which sought to advise the government on the future of health and social care, chaired and led by economist Dame Kate Barker.

Dominic's work with the CPFT included establishing Recovery College East and more recently the trust's Suicide Strategy, which is currently in development, along with its Involvement Strategy. In 2017 he started chairing the Partnership Strategy Group which was tasked with ensuring the Involvement Strategy led to clear, tangible outcomes, such as the Partnership Forum which is currently being established.

Dominic has spoken at various events and has also delivered social media training to staff and patients. He has written a chapter for the book *Ethics from the Ground Up* edited by Dr Julie Wintrup.

Dominic's Twitter handle is @Patient_Leader and he blogs at https://patientleader.wordpress.com.

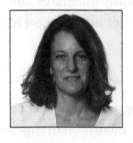 **Sibylle Erdmann** has been working as a parent carer for her two children, both with complex healthcare needs, who are now aged 7 and 9. Her everyday parenting extends to attending hospital appointments, coordinating medical care and advocating for accessibility and inclusion.

Sibylle is passionate about making changes in the here and now, through how we show up and what conversations we have with the people around us. Prior to being a parent carer, she worked in organisational consulting, with topics such as employee voice. She is currently completing her doctorate in organisational change, writing about her lived experience of making healthcare decisions for children. She first became involved in healthcare improvement through UCLPartners and was a founding member of Q, an initiative connecting people who have improvement expertise across the UK, with almost 3000 members today.

Sibylle is a frequent speaker at international healthcare conferences, a member of the BMJ Patient Panel and a BMJ reviewer and contributor. She volunteers with the London Neonatal Operational Delivery Network, chairing the network parent group.

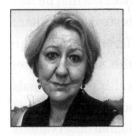 **Alison Cameron's** identity prior to receiving the label 'patient' was her job in international relations. It was not to last. Her colleagues were killed working on one of her projects. What she saw led to her diagnosis of post-traumatic stress disorder and then homelessness, substance misuse and many admissions to hospital.

Once the clouds started to clear, Alison observed where the system was failing people. She resolved to push for change. Now she teaches, writes and speaks at conferences. She was on an Expert Advisory Group to the Department of Health, but her heart is in working with students. When she sees a new member of the NHS Graduate Scheme have a lightbulb moment that might influence how they see patients in the future, it makes the emotional labour worth it.

Alison's blog can be found at https://allywritesblog.wordpress.com.

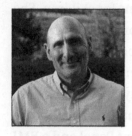

David Festenstein is a communication specialist, coach and professional speaker, who suffered a stroke in 2008 that left him paralysed on his right side and unable to walk. He used a lot of his communication expertise to help him deal with the event and then subsequently to support and drive his recovery process.

During this time David kept an extensive diary and journal that reflected his 'Language of Recovery'. When he reviewed his story and observations, he realised that he had used distinct steps to aid his recovery. His stroke consultant encouraged him to speak at medical conferences, where he got excellent feedback. On the basis of this success, he set up workshops, training and coaching health professionals using his recovery model. The Stroke Association also made a podcast of his story. One of the most valuable observations made about his recovery model is that it can be used for any severe health or personal setback. His recovery model has given many health professionals insights on what they can do further to help their patients in their recovery process.

Some of David's notable speaking engagements have been at the University of Oxford, a global pharmaceutical company in Switzerland, the King's Fund in London and at the Leaders in Healthcare Conference.

For more information about David's speaking, training or coaching programmes please contact him at david@strokerecovery.co.uk.

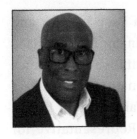 **Patrick Ojeer** is a Patient Leader seeking to transfer services. After one of his sons was born with sickle cell disease, Patrick became aware of the lack of knowledge and management within the NHS for persons with sickle cell disease. He gave up his engineering career to care for his son.

After getting involved with the North West London Managed Network for Haemoglobinopaties as a patient representative, Patrick later became Chair of the NHS London Specialised Commissioning Group Patient and Public Involvement Committee. He was an executive board member of the Sickle Cell Society before being appointed as the interim operations manager of the society. Currently he is a patient representative on the NHS England Specialised Commissioning Clinical Reference Group for Haemaglobinopaties.

Patrick has worked with the NHS National Institute for Health Research Collaboration for Leadership in Applied Health Research and Care Northwest London (NIHR CLAHRC NWL) on the sickle cell GP Education Project, and was project manager on another project, 'Patient Recorded Experience Measure' (PREM) for sickle cell disease. He is a CLAHRC NWL Improvement Leader Fellow and holds an MSc in Improvement Science.

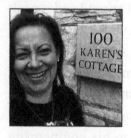

Karen Owen is a Peer Support and Volunteer Co-ordinator for the NHS, a Patient Representative for Thames Valley Clinical Senate, a Patient Partner for Thames Valley Patient Experience, a Patient Representative for Share your Care/Connected Care, a Patient Group Member for Binfield Surgery Patient Group Member, and a member of both HAE UK and Rosamund Snow Community. She actively supports and encourages others to take control of their own destiny and move into patient roles if they feel they can make a difference, on a local, regional and national basis.

Karen's Twitter handle is @GleefulKaz and her blog can be found at https://gleefulkaz.wordpress.com.

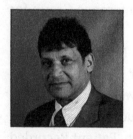

Trevor Fernandes is currently Co-Chair of the East of England Citizens' Senate, which aims to extend the public voice, representing patients with long-term conditions. As a patient living with heart failure, he is motivated by the excellent care he received following two heart attacks and he wants to ensure that everybody has the same opportunity that he had. He is passionate about using his experience as a patient to develop, improve and deliver the best possible outcomes. He continues to work with local and national patient groups to ensure the patient, carer and family perspective is considered in health services.

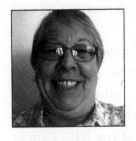

Lesley Preece feels honoured to be amongst the extended community of this extraordinary book. She will be 70 years old when it is published but is stuck at 55, when the accident that took her from her vocation in education occurred. She is a serial failed retiree.

Together with good friend Terry, Lesley has five wonderful adult children – Jennifer, Catherine, David, Harriet and Richard. The family table requires 19 places.

By joining David Gilbert's gang of eight patient partners at Sussex MSK, Lesley has found her tribe, and is holding on fast. She is a NHS-trained mentor.

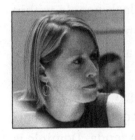

Ceinwen Giles is a founder and Director of Shine Cancer Support, a national charity that supports people in their 20s, 30s and 40s who have experienced a cancer diagnosis. Prior to her work with Shine, she worked for an international development consultancy firm where her clients included the United Nations and the UK's Department for International Development. She has worked as a programme manager in a wide variety of fields including health, community development, and sexual and reproductive rights in countries such as the UK, Canada, Sierra Leone, Vietnam, Thailand and Tanzania.

Ceinwen was diagnosed with stage IV non-Hodgkin lymphoma six weeks after her daughter was born prematurely. She now works with Shine's other founder, staff and trustees to develop Shine's support and information, as well as Shine's fundraising activities.

In addition to her work with Shine, Ceinwen is a Trustee for the Point of Care Foundation, a member of the General Advisory Council of the King's Fund, and a member of the BMJ's patient panel. She is currently interim chair of the Patient and Public Voices Forum for the NHS Cancer Programme.

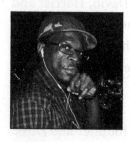 **Dominic Makuvachuma Walker** is an African mental health service user/survivor with a special interest in health service management, research and training. His main focus is on issues specific to Black people within public services, especially the mental health system. Dominic also lives with a range of physical health needs.

After six years as Engagement Manager at Mind, where his portfolio comprised the development of the Peer Support Programme and the Local Influencing Agenda, Dominic is currently an independent consultant, leading the Reigniting the Space project for NSUN.

He has 25 years' experience in supporting the development of lived experience leadership, focusing on health service design and delivery. After a range of engagements including as Joint project lead for the Letting through Light service user led Audits in Birmingham & Ealing, and as an Associate Reviewer with the Health and Social Care Advisory Service Reviewing & evaluating examples of good practice in health service delivery nationally with the Health and Social Care Advisory Service (HASCAS) significantly influenced his views of current mental health services.

Dominic was the first African in England to sit as a panelist on an independent homicide inquiry. He continues to provide training and consultancy for various organisations

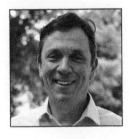

David Gilbert is a mental health service user, writer and poet with 30 years' experience working in healthcare at local, national and international level. He is Patient Director for Sussex MSK Partnership (Central), which was the first such role of its kind in the NHS. He co-founded the Centre for Patient Leadership and NHS Centre for Involvement and is Director of InHealth Associates (www.inhealthassociates.co.uk), which supports patients-as-partners change. He has worked for the Consumers Association, King's Fund, Office for Public Management, Commission for Health Improvement and Croydon PCT. He is Writer in Residence at the Bethlem Gallery, Project Director for RE:CREATE Psychiatry and a visiting lecturer at the University of Hertfordshire. He spends too much time on Twitter (@DavidGilbert43) and on getting upset about Leeds Utd. His blog on all things healthcare and poetry is at https://futurepatientblog.com.

Photographs of David Gilbert and David Festenstein by Mia Festenstein.

FURTHER READING

David Gilbert

Blog: https://futurepatientblog.com

Website: www.inhealthassociates.co.uk

Centre for Patient Leadership, FPM and NHS Midlands and East (2013) 'Bring it on – 40 ways to support Patient Leadership.' http://engagementcycle.org/wp-content/uploads/2013/03/Bring-it-on-40-ways-to-support-Patient-Leadership-FINAL-V-APRIL-2013.pdf

Mark Doughty (2017) 'Talking Leadership – delivering a vision of real collaboration.' *The King's Fund.* https://www.kingsfund.org.uk/publications/articles/mark-doughty-delivering-real-collaboration

David Gilbert (2012) 'The rise of the patient leader.' *Health Service Journal.* https://www.hsj.co.uk/comment/the-rise-of-the-patient-leader/5040463.article

David Gilbert (2017) 'Why we need Patient Leaders.' *British Medical Journal.* https://blogs.bmj.com/bmj/2017/09/21/david-gilbert-why-we-need-patient-leaders

David Gilbert (2017) 'How patient partners are changing healthcare.' *NHS Confederation*. https://www.nhsconfed.org/blog/2017/08/how-patient-partners-are-changing-healthcare

David Gilbert (2018) 'Rethinking Engagement.' *British Journal of Psychiatry 43*, 1, 4–7. https://www.cambridge.org/core/journals/bjpsych-bulletin/article/rethinking-engagement/818554AF0EAB572D47BE9FC29D8CCFA0

David Gilbert (2018) 'The Moonlight World. Digital story about David's mental health experiences and motivation for his Patient Leadership work.' https://www.patientvoices.org.uk/flv/1007pv384.htm

David Gilbert (2018) 'Patient leadership for real: The Sussex model for patient partnership.' *Health Service Journal*. https://www.hsj.co.uk/patient-and-public-involvement/patient-leadership-for-real-the-sussex-model-for-patient-partnership/7022549.article

David Gilbert and Mark Doughty (2012) 'Why patient leaders are the new kids on the block.' *Health Service Journal*. https://www.hsj.co.uk/why-patient-leaders-are-the-new-kids-on-the-block/5046065.article

David Gilbert and Mark Doughty (2013) 'Patient leaders should have been Francis' first recommendation.' *Health Service Journal*. https://www.hsj.co.uk/leadership/patient-leaders-should-have-been-francis-first-recommendation/5061232.article

David Gilbert and Mark Doughty (2013) 'The quiet revolutionaries: patient leaders.' *Health Service Journal*. https://www.hsj.co.uk/leadership/the-quiet-revolutionaries-patient-leaders/5054198.article

David Gilbert and Jeremy Taylor (2016) 'Why patient engagement might have prevented the doctors strike.'

Health Service Journal. https://www.hsj.co.uk/comment/
why-patient-engagement-might-have-prevented-the-doctors-
strike/7001662.article

Becky Seale (2016) 'Patients as Partners: Building collaborative
relationships among professionals, patients, carers and
communities.' *The King's Fund.* https://www.kingsfund.org.
uk/publications/patients-partners

(2016) 'Five minutes with...David Gilbert.' *British Medical
Journal 354.* https://doi.org/10.1136/bmj.i3689

Dominic Stenning

Dominic Stenning (2014) 'It's time to start asking and answering
the hard questions: a view from an expert by experience.'
The King's Fund. https://www.kingsfund.org.uk/blog/2014/04/
its-time-start-asking-and-answering-hard-questions-view-
expert-experience

Dominic Stenning (2019) 'Patients as Leaders: Reflections on
Identity, Equality and Power.' In J. Wintrup *et al.* (eds) *Ethics
from The Ground Up: Emerging debates, changing practices and
new voices in healthcare.* Macmillan International and Red
Globe Press.

Ceinwen Giles

Ceinwen Giles (2014) 'Five tips on how the NHS can work
with patients and the public.' *The Guardian.* https://
www.theguardian.com/healthcare-network/2014/oct/29/
how-nhs-engage-patients-public

Ceinwen Giles (2018) 'How can the NHS work effectively with patients and the public?' *The King's Fund.* https://www.kingsfund.org.uk/blog/2018/04/ nhs-work-effectively-patients-public

Alison Cameron

Blog: https://allywritesblog.wordpress.com/

Alison Cameron (2014) 'Coming out of the box.' *The BMJ Opinion.* https://blogs.bmj.com/bmj/2014/07/17/ alison-cameron-coming-out-of-the-box/ Interview

Alison Cameron (2017) 'Bridging the gap between "them" and "us".' *NHS England Source 4 Networks.* www.source4networks.org.uk/resources/ case-studies/110-spotlight-on-bridge-builders

Alison Moore (2015) 'Interview with Alison Cameron: patient advocate and engagement consultant.' *MiP Health.* https:// www.miphealth.org.uk/home/news-campaigns/Features/ interview-alison-cameron-patient-advocate.aspx

David Festenstein

David Festenstein (2010) 'A Stroke of Luck.' *The Magazine of the Professional Speakers Association.* [available from David on request]

David Festenstein (2013) '7 Steps to Recovery.' *YouTube.* https:// youtu.be/ZfJjaf1u-MM

David Festenstein (2013) 'The Fundamentals of Care.' Talk at The University of Oxford. *YouTube.* https://youtu.be/Gn2lUl6llTk

David Festenstein (2013) 'Stroke Experience.' Lecture at The University of Oxford Brookes. *YouTube*. https://youtu.be/ bsdg_EdYeT4

David Festenstein (2014) 'Quality of Aftercare through the Eyes of a Patient.' *Eye for Pharma*. https://social.eyeforpharma.com/ commercial/quality-aftercare-through-eyes-patient

David Festenstein (2016) 'What does engagement with patients really mean?' Talk at the Leaders in Healthcare Conference. https://www.linkedin.com/pulse/my-presentation-leaders-healthcare-conference-2016-david-festenstein/ also at https:// youtu.be/DNfVqBZJx1Q

W Mitchell, International Keynote Speaker who inspired David Festenstein. For more details go to www.wmitchell.com

Michael Seres

Blog: Beingapatient.blogspot.com

Michael Seres (2014) 'On patient entrepreneurs.' *YouTube*. https:// youtu.be/qRJHBL8GWWE

Michael Seres (2015) 'Healthcare Innovation spotlight: 11.health – what 11H is all about.' *YouTube*. https://youtu.be/ M9hMybMZ8S4

Patrick Ojeer

Aljuburi, G., Okoye, O., Majeed, A., Knight, Y., Green, S.A., Banarsee, R., Nkohkwo, A., Ojeer, P., Ndive, C., Oni, L., Phekoo, K.J. (2012) 'Views of patients about sickle cell disease management in primary care: a questionnaire-based pilot study.' *JRSM Short Reports 3*, 11, 78.

Aljuburi, G., Phekoo, K.J., Okoye, N.O., Anie, K., Green, S.A., Nkohkwo, A., Ojeer, P., Ndive, C., Banarsee, R., Oni, L., Majeed, A. (2012) 'Patients' views on improving sickle cell disease management in primary care: focus group discussion.' *JRSM Short Reports 3*, 12, 1–7.

Chakravorty, S., Tallett, A., Witwicki, C., Hay, H., Mkandawire, C., Ogundipe, A., Ojeer, P., Whitaker, A., Thompson, J., Sizmur, S., Sathyamoorthy, G., Warner, J.O. (2018) 'Patient-reported experience measure in sickle cell disease.' *Archives of Disease in Childhood 10*, 12, 1104–1049.